OTHER BOOKS AND VIDEOS BY KURT BRUNGARDT

THE COMPLETE BOOK OF ABS FOR WOMEN

THE COMPLETE BOOK OF

ABS
FOR WOMEN

THE DEFINITIVE GUIDE FOR WOMEN WHO
WANT TO GET INTO THE ULTIMATE SHAPE

KURT BRUNGARDT

VILLARD NEW YORK

A Villard Books Trade Paperback Original

Copyright © 2004 by Kurt Brungardt

All rights reserved under International and Pan-American Copyright Conventions. Published in the United States by Villard Books, an imprint of The Random House Publishing Group, a division of Random House, Inc., New York, and simultaneously in Canada by Random House of Canada Limited, Toronto.

VILLARD and "V" CIRCLED Design are registered trademarks of Random House, Inc.

LIBRARY OF CONGRESS CATALOGING-IN-PUBLICATION DATA
Brungardt, Kurt.
The complete book of abs for women: the definitive guide for women who want to get into the ultimate shape / Kurt Brungardt.
p. cm.
Includes index.
ISBN 0-8129-6947-2
1. Exercise for women. 2. Abdomen—Muscles. I. Title.

GV482.B78 2004
613.7'045—dc22 2003060028

Villard Books website address: www.villard.com

Printed in the United States of America on acid-free paper

2 4 6 8 9 7 5 3 1

Book design by Mary A. Wirth

This book is dedicated to my mother, Joyce,
and her four sisters—my aunts—whose names also begin with *J*:
Joan, Judy, June, and Jill. They were my biggest influences.

■　■　■

Ab training has been one of the hottest fitness topics for over a decade. Since the publication of *The Complete Book of Abs*, techniques for training the abs have come full circle. Ten years ago, instructors would have discouraged using many of today's popular exercises. Ironically, these new cutting-edge core movements were actually the norm in the 1950s.

This new book brings ab training up to date. Working your abs is about more than just doing crunches; you need to work your entire center—360 degrees around your body. You need to do exercises that train your muscles in isolation and as a functional chain. This book takes what's best from past and current trends and cycles. The routines include traditional isolation exercises and effective movements from Pilates, yoga, and sports training.

The book is also designed for all women, no matter their age or fitness level. It is designed for every stage of a woman's life: from her teenage years to her retirement years. Remember, the key to a healthy lifestyle is to train consistently and intelligently through every phase of your life.

A C K N O W L E D G M E N T S

I decided to be practical and just keep an ongoing list, a thank-you list, not in any particular order, but a combination of how it happened and memory. So here it goes, thanks to

Bruce Tracy, my editor, for making the book a reality, and Adam Korn for all his patience and help.

Dan Strone for his help and support in honing and clarifying ideas. I hope he and Bruce keep having lunch. And Sarah, agent in training, for her help and support and her inspiring abs.

Tracy Marx for all her help with the manuscript and other things.

Doug Stumpf for starting the whole thing.

Mike and Brett, my brothers, for their help and advice.

As always, Debbie and Bryon Holmes for their fitness expertise and the use of their two gyms in Estes Park, Colorado.

Laura Katers for her research, proofreading, and anatomy drawings.

Nate Gross for his boy-type designs.

Robbin Schiff for finding the cover photo and her design.

All the models who posed for the exercises.

Ann Schofield for her generosity in sharing her knowledge and expertise in issues dealing with the transverse abdominis.

New York Sports Club for allowing us to use their gym for all the New York City shoots.

Daron Hays of the Bikram Yoga School in Fort Collins, Colorado, for letting us use his studio and being a great yoga teacher.

Karl Osterbuhr, as the artistic director on all the photo shoots, and for his work in postproduction to get the photos ready.

Definitions Health Club in Denver, Colorado, for letting us use their gym and yoga studio.

CONTENTS

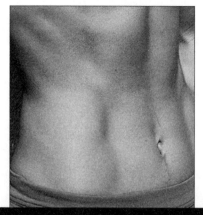

The Foundation

This section will help you set realistic goals and teach you ab train-ing fundamentals, so you can achieve the best results safely and in the least amount of time.

CHAPTER ONE

The First Consultation

PREVIEW: *This chapter is about getting acquainted and discovering how you can best use this book. It will help you organize your time and discover your fitness level and will give you tips for getting started.*

First Session with Your Personal Trainer

The Complete Book of Abs for Women is set up a little differently from most workout books.

Traditionally, exercise books begin with a lot of introductory information before you get into the workouts. All this information is important, but it can also be overwhelming. It can be so overwhelming, in fact, that you give up before you actually start the program. This is primarily a book about doing, about taking action. After reading this chap-

ter and Chapter Two, "Ab Basics," you'll be ready to work out.

In this book, we're going to follow a process that's more like the relationship between a client and her personal trainer. If I were training you and you signed up for ten sessions, I wouldn't spend the first five lecturing you about anatomy, training techniques, and exercise physiology. If I did, you would probably ask for your money back and hire another trainer.

When I train a client, we train on the first day. Then, progressively, step-by-step, we build a program. Along the way, I deliver little monologues that explain the basic elements of anatomy, proper training techniques, and exercise physiology. This happens naturally as issues and questions arise during our workouts. This way, the client becomes grounded in both *practice* (working out) and *theory* (important information and principles). These two elements should organically evolve together.

This is one of the virtues of the personal training process. When you buy a book, you normally get all the information up front, then the workout. By the time you start the workout, you've forgotten most of the information. It's removed from the process of working out. We will follow the personal training model, blending working out with talking.

How to Use This Book

This book was designed to fit your long-term exercise needs. Here are some suggestions on how to use it most effectively:

- Everyone should read Chapter Two, "Ab Basics." This chapter outlines basic techniques that are essential for your success. Even if you're an experienced exerciser, some of these techniques will be new and the rest will be a good review.
- Part Two, "The System," a nine-week ab program, is a great way to jump into this book. Go through all three levels and follow the reading assignments. This applies even if you're an advanced exerciser. You'll master twenty-four exercises, and since it's a new routine, it will add variety to your training. Level One may seem easy, but things progress quickly.

- If you really crave a challenge and you're an advanced trainer with a strong foundation of strength and conditioning, you may start with the Advanced Routine (page 135). Or you may just peruse the routines in Chapter Fifteen and find one that appeals to you.
- If you've given birth within the last six months, you should start with Part Five, "From Baby to Beach."
- This book really is for every stage of a woman's life. This means it's for the whole family. There are routines for kids, teenagers, the over-fifty crowd, and those who want to improve their sports performance.
- As you advance, the instructions in Chapter Sixteen, "Creating Your Own Routine," will show you how to design your own program.
- The book will also get you started on a complete fitness program that includes cardio work, stretching, and weight training.
- Part Three, "The Reader," will coach you through techniques and concepts to help you succeed. These include goal setting, motivation strategies, guidelines to explore your personality and body type, nutrition, and exercise physiology. How you use this book will depend on your goals, fitness level, and lifestyle.

The Relationship: Who Are You?

This is the age-old question when writing a book. Who is my audience? How can I best communicate to them? With a fitness book, this question becomes more specific but is just as mysterious. It can be translated: What are the fitness levels and the goals of my readers? Each reader, of course, will have different answers and will have had varied levels of workout experience.

How would you describe your fitness level? Beginner? Intermediate? Advanced? Are you currently working out? Do you get in the start-and-stop syndrome? How long has it been since you worked out? Will this be your first time on a program? These are questions you need to ask yourself.

GOALS

What are your workout goals? In other words, how much time can you realistically devote to a workout program? The most important element in answering this question is to be brutally honest. We all want everything: a beautiful, healthy body, a satisfying love life, a fulfilling career, loyal friends, a good relationship with our family, a creative outlet, some sort of practice that nurtures our spirit. What I'm saying in a roundabout way is, don't take on more than you can handle. You want a great body and you want it now. But don't take on a workout schedule that's an unrealistic commitment. This is just setting yourself up for failure—and often that's part of a pattern to sabotage yourself.

Maybe, at this point in your life, the only time you can realistically commit to working out is ten minutes in the morning. If this is reality, accept it and fully commit to the ten minutes. You will be rewarded with stronger abdominal and lower-back muscles. This will translate into better posture, more energy, and more confidence in showing off your midriff. If you could also find time for thirty minutes of cardio three times a week, and two weight-training sessions a week, then you would receive even more re-

wards. We'll talk more about a complete program later. But for now, *only set goals you know you can keep*. As you progress, you can increase the challenge if you choose.

TIME

Timewise, when it comes to working out—especially if you're just starting out—it's best to be conservative. It's better to underdo it and stay on the program than to be over-ambitious and quit. Look at it this way: If you were exercising zero minutes a week and you started doing ten minutes four times a week, you'd be doing forty times more than you were. The key to getting started and to achieving your ultimate fitness goals is to be on a program that enables you to exercise consistently over the long haul. And by the long haul, I mean for the rest of your life. It does no good to think, "Oh, I'll work out this year and take next year off." Besides, you want to look and feel good every year.

This book will give you many options—from as little as ten minutes a day to an hour a day.

THE HEALTH FACTOR

The last question is, do you have any specific medical problems or physical limitations? Before doing any of the exercises in this book, you should be 100 percent sure that you are not putting yourself at risk of injury and do not have other health concerns. If done correctly and safely, exercise will improve your body and mind. But you should always check with your doctor before beginning such a program. If you are recovering from an injury or have chronic health problems, make sure you get clearance from your specialist.

Exercise and Monotony

In the famous Greek myth of Sisyphus, Zeus sentenced the king of Corinth to roll a boulder up a hill, only to have it roll back to the bottom every day for the rest of his life. Sisyphus didn't need a day planner, a personal assistant, or voice mail. His was a short list of to-dos. Roll the rock up the hill. Every day, all day long, he rolled the boulder up the hill, only to have it roll back down after he struggled to achieve his goal.

Some people think of ab work as an equally cruel fate. And there are similarities between Sisyphus's ordeal and working out:

• It's physically challenging.
• You need to do it consistently for the rest of your life.
• Repetition is an integral part of working out (although you can find more variety than Sisyphus).

Ultimately, Sisyphus became a hero. He found beauty, integrity, and even a kind of pleasure in the process of rolling the rock up the hill. As you progress and deepen your commitment to wellness, you can become an exercise hero, finding satisfaction in the process of working out, and giving your body a happy, healthy fate. At each fitness level, you will struggle with some of the same dilemmas as Sisyphus.

Reasons to Exercise

Working out and being active are the fountain of youth. Before we get into fitness levels and strategies for using this book, let's look at some important benefits of working out:

• helps keep you slim
• lowers blood pressure
• increases energy levels
• strengthens your heart
• increases sexual pleasure
• improves quality of sleep
• decreases absenteeism at work and school
• speeds recovery time from illness and injury
• improves the efficiency of your cardiovascular system
• increases muscle tone, strength, and flexibility
• slows down the effects of aging

Discovering Your Fitness Levels and Strategies for Using This Book

THE BEGINNER

She's excited and wants results. There are many reasons why she might have decided to start working out. She may see her body losing tone as she moves into her middle twenties. She may have had a baby. As she reaches her thirties, she may want to train in order to stay competitive in her favorite sport. She may want to slow down the aging process as she reaches forty. Or she may just want to get in great shape for the beach.

Strategies for the Beginner

1. For you, the prescription is simple. Just follow the program. If you just had a baby, start the program with Part Five,

"From Baby to Beach" (page 111). Otherwise begin with Level One of the System (page 29).

2. Be patient. It will take at least six weeks before you start to see results.
3. Don't push yourself too hard. It will lead to excessive soreness, which will lead to missing workouts. Unlike Sisyphus, you will not be struck with a thunderbolt if you don't get the rock all the way up the hill.

Guidelines

1. When learning a new movement, practice it while you are fresh: in other words, not when you're exhausted. This can lead to unnecessary frustration.
2. In the beginning, your main focus should be on mastering proper technique. Focus on technique until you can do the movement correctly without thinking, "Is this right?" Instead, you want the voice in your head to give gentle, positive encouragement: "Get my shoulder blades up higher. Keep my head in a good position." When you really know the exercise, you can coach yourself.

THE COMEBACK KID

She's coming back after a long layoff, more than a year. This layoff could have been because of an injury, a baby, or just laziness. Every day is a battle against sloth. Whatever the reason, she's back!

Strategies for the Comeback Kid

1. Start with Level One of the System and work your way through the program. If you just had a baby, start with Part Five, "From Baby to Beach."
2. Unlike the beginner, you are going to

have some muscle memory and you will have done some of the exercises before. But don't let your ego get in the way and try to get back to your old form too quickly. Although your mind will want to jump ahead, your body needs to move at the pace of a beginner. Your mind might think it can roll the rock all the way up the hill without any negative consequences on the body, but this is a myth of the mind. So go slow and steady and work your way through the System.

Guidelines

1. Stick with the pace of the program and don't be impatient and try to move forward too fast.
2. Even if you think you know the exercise, review the instructions and Trainer's Tips before you jump into it.

THE STRUGGLER

She's in the middle of the pack, not a beginner or an advanced fitness Superwoman. She wants to be fit and healthy, but she struggles to stay on a consistent program. She is stuck in the hellish limbo of the start-and-stop syndrome. She's done workout tapes, taken classes, joined a gym, and probably bought a piece of fitness equipment (that's now in the closet); she reads health and fitness magazines (at least leafs through them on the stands), and there's a good chance she's purchased an exercise book. She stays with a workout for a while, then quits exercising for a few months.

The Struggler intimately understands the fate of Sisyphus. She feels the weight and boredom of rolling the rock and eventually, metaphorically, gets rolled over and takes a seat at the bottom of the mountain. She was once a beginner and has had a glory day or two as an exercise hero. Like all of us, she wants the best fate for her body.

Strategies for the Struggler

1. Stay simple and start with Part Two, "The System," and go through all three levels. Level One may seem easy, but it will help build a foundation and create the exercise habit without creating stress.
2. Work at your own pace and add the other fitness elements—cardio, weights, and stretching—to your program.
3. When you feel the rock becoming a task too much to bear, for whatever reason, change up your program. Go to Part Six, "The Routines," and pick a routine that seems fun. You have an advantage over Sisyphus. You have free will to create variety anytime you choose.
4. After you've trained for three months straight, give yourself a break—take a few days off. The important thing is that you consciously choose the break. You're not giving up. Taking these breaks will be the very thing that allows you to come back and train at a higher level. It will also allow you to keep training over the long haul.

Guidelines

1. You need to make a commitment to a program long-term. Chapter Seven will help you set these long-term goals.
2. Set realistic goals. Even if you'd like to do more, stay realistic. Starting and stopping often boils down to trying to do too much. Then "I don't have enough time" becomes an excuse to quit.
3. Find ways to motivate and challenge

yourself when you teeter on quitting. Hire a personal trainer for a month. Do whatever it takes.

THE SUPERWOMAN

She has made fitness an important and integral part of her lifestyle. She has been working out consistently for at least two years. Rolling the rock up the hill has been transformed from a chore to a kind of pleasure. She's an exercise hero.

Strategies for the Superwoman

1. There are many ways this book can challenge you if you're a Superwoman. You can go through Part Two, "The System," but add weight to the movements so your repetitions stay in the prescribed range.
2. You could start with Level Three of the System.
3. You could start with the Advanced Routine (page 135) in Chapter Fifteen.
4. You could do any of the specialized routines to challenge your abdominals and inner core, adding variety and excitement to your training.

Guidelines

1. At this level, your challenge is to harness the power of the mind (the mind-muscle link) while maintaining perfect technique.
2. You need to continually find new ways to motivate and challenge yourself with a complete program that includes weight training, cardio, and stretching. Also challenge yourself to keep your intensity levels high.
3. Don't overtrain and/or become too self-critical. This takes the joy and pleasure out of working out.

4. Look at Chapter Sixteen, "Creating Your Own Routine," to incorporate advanced principles into your program.

Getting Started: When and Where

An important step in getting started is deciding when and where you want to train. If you aren't specific about this, you'll keep finding a way to put it off until the day is gone and the rock is still untouched.

When. Set a specific time each day when you are going to work out. One time is not necessarily better than another. It just depends on your schedule. It could be in the morning or before you go to bed. Just don't do it right after you eat. Give yourself a couple of hours to digest.

Where. Know where you are going to train. If it's at home, choose a spot where you can spread out your mat and have the least interruptions. Create your own little home gym. If you train at a gym, then the answer is obvious.

When and where are important in creating the habit, the ritual. It is like setting up a date for yourself. Don't stand yourself up.

CHAPTER TWO

Ab Basics

PREVIEW: *This chapter will introduce you to the key concepts, techniques, and principles of abdominal training. You will acquire a basic understanding of anatomy and learn fundamental, but often neglected, exercise techniques that are essential for safety and achieving the best results.*

Your Exercise Anatomy

A BODY OF KNOWLEDGE

As a trainer, one of the things I've noticed about my female clients is their openness to talk about and understand their bodies in a new way. Women have always been ahead of men when it comes to relating to their bodies. Self-care books for women become bestsellers. These books are practically nonexistent for men. Getting in touch with your anatomy is an important part of the exercise process. The goal of this con-

versation is not to make you an anatomy professor, but to simply introduce you to the basic muscles. It's a get-to-know-yourself session designed to help you learn some names and locations. Knowing these names and locations will help you visualize and communicate with your abs during your workout.

The Rectus Abdominis

You all know the rectus abdominis. It's the famous "six-pack," the rippling washboard. Anatomically, the rectus is one long sheath

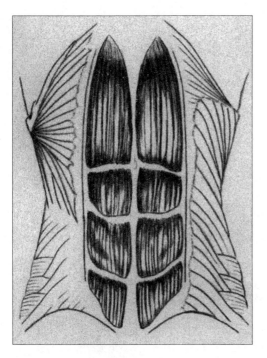

of muscle that runs from your sternum (breastbone) to your pubic bone.

Abdominal Biomechanics

The main function of the rectus in ab work is flexion, bending your torso forward. It shortens the distance between your hips and chest. It also acts as a stabilizing muscle in other movements. When it comes to doing ab work, your rectus abdominis will function in three basic ways:

1. It will move your chest (breastbone) toward your hips (pubic bone).
2. It will move your hips (pubic bone) toward your chest (breastbone).
3. It will simultaneously move your chest (breastbone) and your hips (pubic bone) toward each other.

The following exercises use the rectus abdominus.

Exercise Examples

The Crunch. When you do a crunch, you curl your chest toward your hips. If your upper body is initiating the movement (as in a crunch), then you will feel more stress in the upper area of the rectus abdominis. (See photos on page 188.)

Reverse Crunch. When you do a reverse crunch, you move your hips toward your chest. Since the movement is initiated from your hips (lower body), you will feel more stress in your lower abs. (See photos on page 160.)

Double Crunch. In this movement, you simultaneously bring your hips and chest together. Since the movement is initiated from both your hips and your chest, you are working both your upper and your lower abs equally. (See photos on page 205.)

Rule of thumb: Whenever you move your chest toward your hips or your hips toward your chest, you are working your rectus abdominis. Now you can communicate with that muscle. You can take this knowledge into any class or workout and know where to focus, even if the instructor isn't explaining which area you're working.

The Upper/Lower Abs Controversy

Anatomically there are no such things as upper and lower abs. As I explained above, and as the illustration on this page shows, the rectus abdominis is one long sheath of muscle that runs from the breastbone to the pubic bone. It is also attached to the fifth, sixth, and seventh ribs on each side of your rib cage. So when you do a movement that activates the rectus, the entire rectus gets activated. So why upper and lower abs?

Let me give you an example from the world of fashion. Let's take the term *waist*. Where is your waist? It's a trick question. Your waist is nowhere. It doesn't exist. You will not find it in any anatomy book. You can't break your waist like a bone or pull your waist like a muscle. *Waist* is a term made up by the fashion industry. Even though it doesn't exist anatomically, it's a very useful idea for a clothing designer. In the same way, the idea of upper and lower abs can be very useful to you as an exerciser.

This is what I call creative anatomy. Looking at the body from a strictly literal perspective is essential if you're writing an anatomy textbook or a medical text for doctors. You don't want surgeons searching in vain for the lower abs in the middle of an operation. When you're exercising, however, it is helpful to be creative and to focus your mind specifically on a target area. Upper and lower ab areas give your mind more specific places on which to focus.

When I work out, I can feel the different movements putting emphasis on different areas of my rectus abdominis. I am not the only one to have discovered this. Classic books like *Legendary Abs* use this breakdown. Countless numbers of professional bodybuilders, athletes, and personal trainers employ this breakdown when they train.

The old stereotypical professor who has spent a lifetime in the classroom and not in the gym may waggle his or her finger at you and say, "My dear, the rectus abdominis is one sheath of muscle that runs from your pubic bone to your sternum." You can nod yes because you know the facts. You also know that exercise is an act of creativity where the mind and body fuse.

For these reasons, we will think about the rectus as having upper and lower regions, like the north and south of a country. And since free choice is important and everyone is different, if you want to think of the rectus as strictly one muscle, this is okay, too. Do what is most helpful to you.

The Infamous Obliques

The obliques—aka the "love handles"—wrap around your sides and act as a frame for the rectus abdominis. Now let's get more specific. There are two sets of obliques: external and internal.

External Obliques. The external obliques originate from the lower eight ribs and move diagonally down, inserting at the front half of the hip on the crest of the ilium, which is the top of the hipbone. They are also attached to the rectus abdominis and the serratus muscle that covers the ribs.

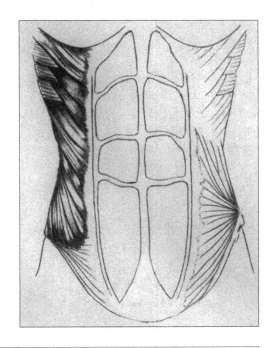

Internal Obliques. The internal obliques originate at the crest of the ilium—the top of the hip—and travel diagonally upward, crisscrossing the external obliques and inserting on the eighth, ninth, and tenth ribs. They are also attached to the lower-back

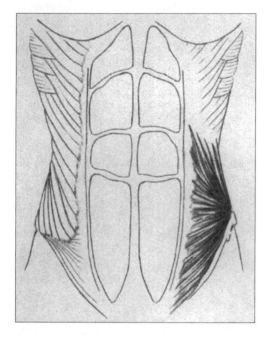

muscles and the rectus abdominis. The internal obliques are underneath the external obliques.

Abdominal Biomechanics
You use your obliques whenever you twist, rotate, or bend at the waist.

Exercise Examples

Crunch with a Twist. In this exercise, when the right shoulder is crossing toward the left knee, you are activating the oblique muscles. (See photos on page 207.)

Bent-Knee Leg-Overs. In this exercise, your obliques are rotating the hips from side to side. (See photos on page 182.)

Lying Side Bends. In this exercise, as the rib cage bends toward the side of the hip, you are activating the obliques. (See photos on page 184.)

Rule of thumb: So, whenever you twist your torso or hips or bend to your side, you are working your obliques. Now you can communicate with your obliques in any exercise situation, putting your mind on the muscle.

The Hidden and Forgotten Transverse Abdominis
The major ab muscles are built in layers. On top are the rectus abdominis and the external obliques. The internal obliques are located underneath the external obliques, and the transverse abdominis runs horizon-

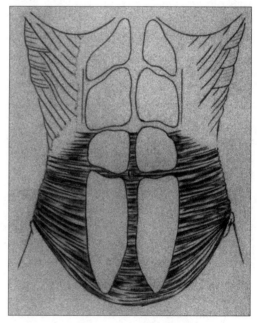

tally underneath all three muscle groups. It is a deep, internal muscle. Since the transverse abdominis isn't a sexy external muscle, it often gets overlooked. But it helps give your abs a sleek, long look. It's a very important player in the overall appearance of your midsection and the strength of your core.

Abdominal Biomechanics

The transverse abdominis pulls the abdominal wall inward and upward. It helps give your entire core area structural support, and it helps stabilize your spine. This is important for proper organ function and good posture. It is an inner girdle of support for your center. When you bring your navel toward your spine, for example, it is the transverse abdominis that is initiating this movement.

Exercise Example

Vacuum Pump. This exercise isolates the transverse abdominis by pulling it up and in. (See photos on page 225.)

Rule of thumb: Whenever you pull your abdomen toward your spine, you are activating your transverse abdominis.

PUTTING IT INTO PRACTICE

Your major abdominal muscles are a masterful design of crisscrossing layers that create a web of support for movement, balance, and stability. Now that you know the abdominal muscles you'll be working, you can start to put this knowledge into action in your workouts. This knowledge will allow you to put your mind on a particular muscle when you're exercising. This mental focus is what makes all the difference between a good workout and a great workout.

Basic Training Principles

GETTING OFF TO A GOOD START

As you start on the System and begin to look over the first routine, keep the following principles in mind.

Mastering the Technique. In the beginning, it is essential to master the proper technique for each exercise. This is the first step; everything else takes a backseat. Don't worry about the recommended reps for each exercise; this is secondary. It doesn't matter how many reps you do if you're doing them wrong. When learning a new exercise, do it when you're fresh. You need to allow a little extra time to study the photos and read the instructions. You need to get a sense of the overall movement as well as the finer points of the exercise.

Adding Intensity. Once you have mastered proper technique, then you can start to push yourself harder. If you haven't mastered proper technique and you try to push it, you increase your risk of injury.

A Breakdown in Technique. A question for many clients is, "When do I stop doing an exercise?" The questions always linger: "Could I have done one more? Was I really tired?" The simplest criterion is a breakdown in technique. This means when you can no longer do the exercise properly, it is time to stop. Let's say you're doing a crunch and you have to pull your neck forward to get your shoulder blades off the ground—that's a breakdown in technique. When your technique gets sloppy, you're no longer working the targeted area. That means it's time to stop.

WARMING UP

It is important to warm up your body before you start exercising. Warming up will do three important things:

1. Increase blood flow to the muscles, allowing them to work more efficiently.
2. Increase muscle temperature, allowing the muscles to contract more forcefully and with more speed. In other words, your workouts will be more intense.
3. Reduce your chance of injury.

Move the Body. Even if you're just doing ab work, you should warm your body up and prepare the areas you're going to work.

• Warm up with five minutes of light aerobic work or increased activity. The activity can be functional, such as any household chore where you turn and twist and move your body, or it can be fun, such as playing with or walking your dog.
• Next, prepare the areas you're going to use with the Stretching Routine (page 96).

FULL RANGE OF MOTION: A ONE, A TWO, AND A THREE

It is essential to perform all exercises through their full range of motion and to keep resistance on the muscles throughout the entire movement. The range of motion will vary from exercise to exercise.

SPEED OF MOVEMENT

As a general rule, you want to keep the speed slow and controlled throughout the entire range of motion. This keeps tension on the ab muscles and doesn't let gravity and momentum do the work instead of your abs.

As you get more advanced, you may choose to vary the speed to create variety or to train for sports-specific movements.

RESTING

The purpose of rest time is to let your muscles recover for the next set. Many variables determine how long you should rest between ab exercises. In the System, your rest time is set for you. But since everyone comes to the program at a different fitness level, you may need to rest between exercises. In general, with ab work, you try to limit your rest between exercises, moving directly from exercise to exercise. Here are some exceptions to this rule:

• If you're a beginner, you may need more rest time.
• If you're doing an advanced routine with weight, then you need to rest between exercises.
• If you're doing athletic explosive movements, you'll also need recovery time.

Basic Techniques

BREATHING

Breathing when you're exercising or doing any activity is essential in order to stay energized and efficient in your movements. Okay, so you know you have to breathe. I know I'm supposed to breathe, too, but I still catch myself holding my breath when I work out. I have to constantly remind myself. That's why in yoga class the instructor reminds you in every posture to breathe. During exercise, the rule of thumb is to exhale during the working portion of the exercise. By working portion, I mean when you are moving against the most resistance. You should inhale when you're moving against the least resistance, to refuel by bringing in fresh oxygen.

Let's put this principle into an exercise situation. If you're doing a crunch, you are moving against the most resistance when you are raising your torso off the floor, going against the force of gravity. This is when you would exhale. As you lower your body back down, you are moving against less resistance, so you would inhale.

Let's look at a non-ab example, since you'll be strength-training soon. If you're doing a bicep curl, when you're curling the weight up, you are moving against the most resistance, so you would exhale. When you're lowering the weight, you are moving against less resistance, so you would inhale.

One caveat when it comes to ab work: Since the movements are small, sometimes it's hard to stay with this strict breathing form. If you're struggling, then try to breathe in a rhythm that supports your body's movement. Most important, *don't hold your breath!*

HEAD AND HAND POSITIONS

Proper Head Position
It's important that you maintain the correct head position when you do ab work. Proper head position will give the best results and help prevent injury.

Guidelines

Chin and Chest Rule. During most ab movements, you want to have about a fist's dis-

tance between your chin and chest. For some people, it helps to think of holding an apple or a tennis ball between their chest and chin.

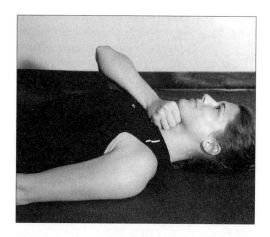

Lengthen Your Neck. In some positions, such as reverse crunches and leg lifts, your head will be resting on the floor or slightly raised. In these positions, you want to keep your neck lengthened and not arched. This may fatigue your neck, so support your head with you hand(s) if the exercise allows. Eventually, your neck will get stronger and this won't be an issue. That's a side benefit

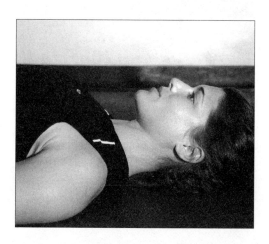

of ab work—it strengthens your neck. Your spine needs to be strong from top to bottom.

You don't want to unnaturally arch your neck.

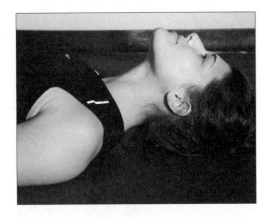

The Towel. If this puts too much stress on your neck, you can place a towel underneath your head.

You can also place a towel under your chin.

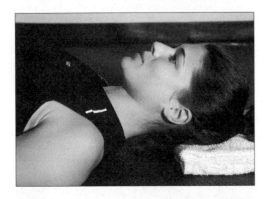

Neck Strain

Doing ab work can put a little extra stress on your neck. Don't blame this on your abs; they're innocent. It's the weight of your head. Your head weighs between seven and ten pounds, so when you have to hold it up during ab work, it puts a lot of extra stress

on the neck. To alleviate the neck pain, you need to focus on the problem child—your head. The way to do this is to support the weight of your head with your hands. This takes the stress off your neck and puts it on your shoulders and arms. Here are some options:

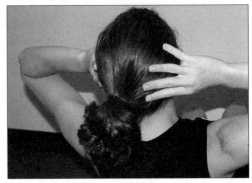

Both Hands Behind Head. Support your head behind your ears with your fingertips. This takes the stress off the neck. But you still have to make the mental shift, allowing the shoulders and arms to do the work. We are conditioned to use the neck to hold up the head. You will need to consciously give your neck muscles the message to relax. They will quickly learn to trust your hands.

A *common mistake* is to interlace your fingers and pull your head forward, driving

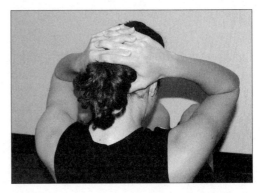

your chin toward your chest. This can hurt your neck and it also limits the range of motion through which your abdominal muscles can work.

One Hand. Another option is to support your head with just one hand. Again, you'll have to give your neck the message to relax, so your hand, shoulder, and arm can do the work.

The Towel. You can also use a towel to support your head. Place the towel behind your head and hold the ends with each hand. It helps to spread the towel out, creating a web of support for the back of your head.

DEFINITIONS

Repetition: A repetition is the completion of one entire movement in an exercise. One repetition of a crunch would be curling your upper body off the mat and lowering it back to the floor. That would equal one repetition. If you did that movement ten times, that would be ten repetitions. (You probably knew that.) Repetitions are also referred to as reps.

Set: A set is the completion of one or more repetitions. If your goal was to do ten repetitions and you did ten, that would be one set of ten reps. If you did just nine reps, you still did a set, even though you didn't quite reach your goal. It would just mean you did one set of nine reps.

Peak Contraction: This is the contraction (tensing or shortening) of the working muscle at the peak of the movement. In a crunch, the peak of the movement is when you've raised your shoulder blades off the floor and you haven't begun to lower your shoulder blades back to the floor.

Hand Positions

Different hand positions can make an exercise easier or more difficult. In general, the farther you place the weight of your arms from your center, the more difficult the exercise will be. This is also true if you're adding weight to the exercise with a dumbbell or weight plate. Let's look at some examples:

Hands Extended. In this position, you can't support your head, but you are decreasing the workload on your abs. The forward position of your arms places the weight of your arms over the center of your body, making most movements easier.

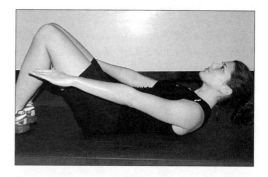

Hands Across Chest. This intermediate position shifts the weight of your arms back toward your torso, increasing the load.

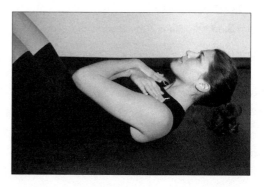

Both Hands Behind Head. This position moves the weight of your arms even farther from your center, increasing the difficulty even more.

These choices give you options for adjusting the workout intensity for different exercises.

Creative Use of Hand Positions

Let's say you were doing crunches and your goal was twelve repetitions. On your tenth rep, you're near your exhaustion point, so you switch your hands from behind your head to across your chest, which allows you to push out another repetition. Then, for the last rep, you extend your hands out and miraculously get that last rep.

WEIGHT RESISTANCE: INCREASING THE INTENSITY

Adding light weights to ab exercises is a way to increase intensity while staying within the recommended repetitions.

Using weight is an advanced technique, so don't do it until you've progressed through all the levels of the System or unless you're an advanced exerciser. In ab work, a little weight means a lot. Start out by adding just two and a half pounds. This may not seem like much, but if you maintain proper technique and isolate the abs, you will feel the difference. The tendency when adding weight to ab work is to recruit other muscles and to use momentum instead of isolating the abs. So start light and keep your technique strict.

You can add weight resistance on almost any ab exercise. This is normally done with the use of weight plates, dumbbells, ankle weights, or a medicine ball.

Upper Body

The safest way to add weight for upper-body movements is to place a weight across your chest. The photo below shows weight added to a crunch.

A SIMPLE NECK STRENGTHENER

Don't worry, this exercise won't give you a big thick neck like a football player's. But it will strengthen the neck muscles that support your head in ab work. Here's the drill:

• Lie on a weight bench or on your bed so your head and neck hang off the edge with no support.
• From this position, use your neck muscles to hold and stabilize your head level with your spine in the same position as if you were standing. It is the same lengthened neck you want in ab work—with a fist's distance between your chin and chest.

PLAN OF ACTION

• Start off with a five-second hold, then, at your own pace, increase the hold by five seconds until you reach a sixty-second hold. You may be able to add five seconds each session. Or it may take a few sessions before you're ready to add on time.
• Do this exercise twice a week.
• If you do it on your ab day, do it after your ab workout or at a different time.

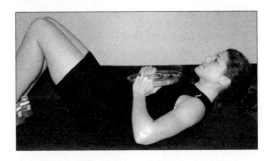

Lower Body

For movements that involve the lower body, you have two choices: holding the weight between your feet or holding a medicine ball between your knees.

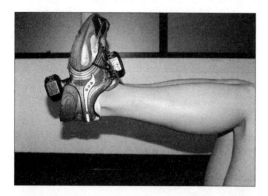

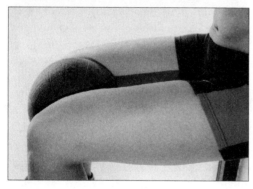

GETTING IN TOUCH WITH YOUR INNER CORE

Most of the time, when we work our abs, we just focus on the famous big outer muscles: the six-pack muscle (rectus abdominis) and the love handles (obliques). We neglect our deep inner muscles, the pelvic floor and the transverse abdominis. These muscles support your center like a natural girdle or a weight belt. If these inner muscles are weak, regardless of how strong your big external muscles are, you will still be vul-nerable to injury, and your body will not function at peak efficiency. So it is essential that you train your inner and outer muscles. When you set your center, you get these deeper muscles prepared to exercise. We need to take a closer look at these deep inner muscles that stabilize and support your spine.

Activating Your Pelvic Floor

The pelvic floor is the area you exercise when you do Kegels. This web or sling of fascia extends from the front of your pelvis to your lower spine, surrounding your vaginal, urethral, and rectal openings. It is like a thin hammock of support. The classic way to get in touch with your pelvic floor is during urination. As you're urinating, bring the stream to a stop. Eureka, that's your pelvic floor shutting down the flow. Before you start to exercise, you want to activate this muscle group. You don't want to give it the death-grip squeeze, just a little squeeze to activate it for inner support.

Engaging Your Transverse Abdominis

As I explained in the exercise anatomy section, your transverse abdominis is the deep muscle that runs horizontally across your midsection. It wraps around your waist like a corset and pulls your abdominal wall in, stabilizing your spine. When your abdomen bulges out, you've lost contact with your transverse abdominis. You can activate your transverse abdominis by drawing your belly button toward your spine. It is important to initiate this engagement down low at your navel level. Otherwise, you will be using your rectus abdominis to execute the movement. The idea is to gently lower your belly button, primarily engaging your transverse abdominis.

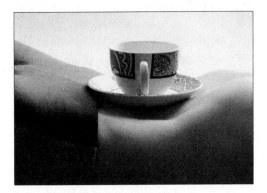

Choice of Engagement

When activating your inner core, you need to experiment to find what works best for you. Research shows that if you activate either your pelvic floor muscles or your transverse abdominis, the other one will also engage. It is easier for me to activate my pelvic floor and then feel my transverse abdominis automatically tighten with ease. Starting with my pelvic floor also helps me keep the focus in my lower abs. But you should experiment and find out what works best for you.

SORENESS

Muscle soreness is common after a workout. Don't worry if you're a little sore (good pain). Soreness is the result of microscopic tears in the muscle. They need recuperation time to repair. If you are too sore to train in your next session, you've overdone it. Most of the time, it is good to train through mild soreness. The increased blood flow in the area will help repair the tissue.

How Hard Do You Squeeze?

Another important element in activating and cinching up your inner-core muscles is getting in touch with the level of intensity you should use to contract them. Ann Schofield, a physical therapist at Colorado State University who specializes in inner-core training, says, "You should contract the muscles at about 30 percent of their maximum. Or a 3 on a scale of 10. You don't want to give them a death squeeze." If you squeeze them too intensely, you'll wear them out and they won't be able to give you support throughout the day or during a long workout.

Cinch and Synch

One of the challenges is getting a feel for all of this. I like to think of the words *cinch* and *synch*. The word *cinch* has two meanings. It means to draw in or tighten. It also means a thing done with ease, as in the phrase, "It's a cinch." Tightening with ease is a key element in activating your inner core. This cinching movement is not simply sucking in your gut, which activates your rectus abdominis and causes your spine to bend slightly forward. Instead you want to—with ease—draw your lower abs in from your pubic bone to your navel. The ultimate goal behind cinching up the inner core is to enable it to work in synch with your bigger external muscles, like the rectus abdominis and obliques, and to work with your arms and legs in everyday activities, as well as in complicated athletic movements. So, cinch and synch.

To Sum Up

The inner core is made up of the deeper muscles that are closer to your spine. These aren't as famous as the six-pack muscle or the love handles, but they are every bit as important. The deep inner muscles that we are most concerned with are the pelvic floor muscles and the transverse abdominis. Now that you know how to get in touch with these muscles, you'll be able to integrate them into the protocol that follows.

The Protocol

PHASE ONE: THE BEGINNING

Let's look in detail at the proper starting position for the center of your body. Setting the center literally means getting the middle of your body ready to work. The first step in this process of finding your "neutral" spine is like finding the balance point in a teeter-totter. When a teeter-totter is balanced, neither end is pointing up or down. It is balanced in the level position. In neutral, your pelvis is also level. Let's try to make this concrete.

One way to explore neutral is to move through both extremes. Lie flat on your back and tilt your pelvis forward, increasing the curve in your back.

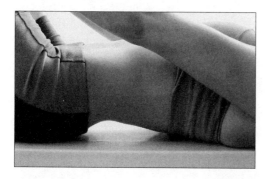

Now tilt your pelvis backward, rounding your back against the floor.

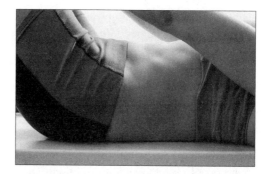

Now let your pelvis rest in the middle, balanced between these two extremes. Then let your pelvis naturally relax down toward the floor, so there is a thin space between your lower back and the floor. This is neutral.

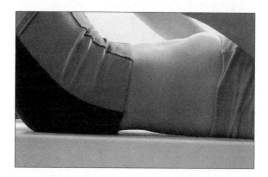

Another way is to rest your hands on your pelvis, pointing your fingers toward your feet. If you're in neutral, your hands should be level, as if they were resting on a tabletop. Theoretically, you could rest a glass of water on your hands and the waterline would be level.

If the imaginary waterline is tilting toward your feet like it might spill in that direction, or your fingers are angled down, then your pelvis is tilted forward.

If the imaginary waterline is tilting back like it could spill on your belly, or your fingers are angled up, then your pelvis is tilted backward.

The goal of a neutral spine is to set the correct and natural relationship between your pelvis and your lower spine before you start exercising. You want the spine to maintain its natural curve and not be unnaturally flattened or curved.

As you relax your lower back and engage your transverse abdominis by bringing your navel toward your spine, your lower back may make light contact with the floor. During some exercise movements, like the curling motion of a crunch, it will also naturally round to the floor. This is okay.

If you feel like you need to slightly tuck your pelvis so your lower back touches the floor for support, this is okay. Eventually, the goal is a neutral spine. Just don't force your lower back to the floor with an unnatural backward tilt of your pelvis.

You need to always be careful of movements that cause your pelvis to unnaturally tilt forward, creating an exaggerated arch in your lower back. This often happens when doing leg lifts. As you lower your feet close to the floor, your lower back arches to compensate, pulling you out of neutral and putting your lower back in danger.

Instead, let your neutral spine determine your range of motion. Only lower your legs to move within a range that allows your pelvis to stay in a safe neutral position. It will be different for everyone. With improved ab and lower-back strength, your range of motion will eventually increase.

GOOD PAIN VERSUS BAD PAIN

You're not going to get to a new and better place without being challenged and pushing yourself. When you're working out, you are going to have to push yourself through some discomfort. As a woman, because of childbirth, you are hardwired to deal with this better than a man. When you're pushing yourself through the last repetition, causing your muscles to adapt and grow stronger, you need to be able to tell the difference between good pain and bad pain. You want to challenge yourself, not injure yourself.

Good pain is that feeling of being pumped, the good burn of fatiguing the muscle. Eventually, you will naturally push to this point, you will thrive in the burn, learn to love it (in a certain way). It's that feeling that is expressed in the phrase, "I had a great workout!"

Bad pain is a warning sign that says, "Stop! Don't push!" Warning signs include shooting pains, sharp pains, and spasms. Whenever pain moves beyond the area you're working, that is a sign to stop and evaluate. Bad pain is an indication that you've injured yourself or are putting yourself in danger.

Train hard; train smart.

PHASE TWO: MOVING THROUGH THE MIDDLE

Now let's get back to the exercise movement. Phase Two of our exercise protocol, the middle phase, is moving from the starting position and returning back to the starting position. In other words, it is everything that happens between the start and the finish.

The first half of this phase is moving toward the position of your peak contraction. In a crunch, this would be as you curl forward, bringing your shoulder blades off the ground.

The second half of this phase is returning at a controlled speed back to the starting position. In a crunch, this would be lowering your shoulder blades back to the floor.

The key elements in this phase are

- keeping the movement slow and controlled
- keeping the movement fluid
- pausing at the moment of peak contraction
- keeping your mind focused on the working muscle(s)

PHASE THREE: THE FINISH

You have to always finish strong. This means not resting at the bottom of the movement and relaxing into the floor. In doing a crunch, let your shoulder blades just lightly touch the floor, maintaining the integrity of your starting position—the neutral spine and an activated inner core—then, of course, start your next repetition.

This beginning, middle, and finish make the progression of each rep. Then, on the next rep, the story starts again.

Remember, *focus your mind* on the muscle and the movement, keeping the motion controlled and fluid.

TO SUM UP

This protocol will become second nature with practice. It will take just a second or two to get focused and start moving the right way. Right now, we're breaking things down into steps and being very specific. But it will pay off in the long run. This procedure guarantees that you activate the right muscles in the right order. It ensures that you engage the smaller deep muscles first. For your body to function at peak efficiency, the smaller, deep inner muscles and the bigger external muscles need to work as a team.

A CASE STUDY: THE ART OF THE SET

When it comes to working out, quality is more important than quantity. This is true when it comes to doing each repetition and when it comes to doing your entire set. We looked in detail at how each rep has a beginning, a middle, and an end. The same is true of a set.

Every set is a cumulative build to failure. So, just because your first repetitions are easy doesn't mean you can just phone them in. You need to strive for quality in each repetition, incorporating all of the protocol.

Let's say your goal for a set is twelve repetitions. You're moving along one quality rep after another. Then around rep seven, you start to feel the fatigue and burn. You stay focused on proper technique and work through the good pain on reps eight and nine. On rep ten, you really struggle and squeeze it out.

Now let's slow things down, as we're coming to that dramatic moment—the moment of failure. This moment boils down to one of the most frequently asked questions: "When should I stop the exercise?" There's always that nagging voice saying, "I could have done a few more." The clearest answer is this: Stop when you have a breakdown in technique. Now let's go back to the exercise, on the eleventh rep.

On rep eleven of your crunch, you let the entire weight of your body give in to the floor, using the floor to push off, and pull your head forward to help curl your torso up. These are all signs that the set is over—you've had a breakdown in technique and you're no longer executing quality repetitions and receiving the benefits of the exercise. Here are the reasons:

- By giving your weight into the floor, you're taking the tension off the working muscle(s).
- By pushing off the floor, you're using momentum and other muscles instead of your abs to execute the movement.
- By pulling on your head, you're trying to use your body to gain a mechanical advantage to help you do the movement. This not only takes the tension off the working muscle(s), but also puts you at risk of injury.

TRAINER'S TIPS

At the end of each exercise description is a list of Trainer's Tips. These have the dual purpose of acting as reminders and giving exercise-specific advice. The following tips could be applied to almost any exercise:

1. Maintain proper head position.
2. Keep your pelvis in neutral.
3. Engage your inner core before each movement.
4. Hold a peak contraction at the top of the movement.
5. Control both the up and down phases of the movement, keeping constant tension on the working muscle(s).
6. Focus your mind on the working muscle(s).
7. Work through the good pain, but when you have a breakdown in technique, stop.
8. Keep the motion fluid.

THE IDEAL WORKOUT

The following is a template of an ideal ab workout.

1. Warm up.
2. Prepare the neck and lower back with a few stretches.
3. Focus on your breathing, bringing your mind and body to the present moment.
4. Visualization One: Create a snapshot in your mind's eye of the abs you want.
5. Shake out your body and repeat a Self-Talk phrase (page 000) a few times to get psyched up.
6. Stay focused, keeping the mind-muscle link throughout your workout.
7. Activate your inner core.
8. Perform each rep in a fluid and controlled manner.
9. Hold your peak contraction.
10. Breathe.
11. Make the whole routine like a dance.
12. Cool down using controlled breathing to center your body.
13. Visualization Two: Hold the ideal snapshot in your mind for a moment as you feel your abs merging with the image.
14. Shake it out, take a deep breath, and let it go, allowing your unconscious mind to work on it.
15. Congratulate yourself on completing your workout.

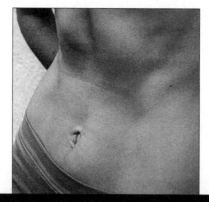

PART TWO

The System

The System is a progressive nine-week ab program that incorporates the latest training techniques to strengthen and tone your abs, lower back, and deep core muscles.

The System has three levels:

1. LEVEL ONE (BEGINNER)

2. LEVEL TWO (INTERMEDIATE)

3. LEVEL THREE (ADVANCED)

It is designed to work interactively with chapters that are assigned from Part Three, "The Reader." These two sections will help your mind and body work together to achieve your goals.

CHAPTER THREE

The System: Level One

REQUIRED READING:
CHAPTER SIX, "THE BODY"

How the System Is Designed

The System combines two abdominal-training philosophies: traditional exercises based on the concept of isolation, and core or functional movements. Routine One, the Traditional Routine, isolates the muscles using exercises that you are familiar with, such as crunches. Routine Two, the Func-tional Routine, trains your center 360 degrees around your body. It uses exercises you may not be so familiar with, such as planks. In tandem, these routines will give you a complete abdominal-training system.

Pep Talk

Okay, it's time for the first workout. Don't panic—there's always going to be a learning curve when you embark on a new project. Embrace the learning curve, love the learning curve—love your own curves. In the beginning, the most important thing is to focus on learning how to do the exercises properly. Don't get frustrated if the movements feel awkward at first. What is important is that you make a little progress each workout.

Goals

The ultimate goal of Level One is to get to Level Two. The fitness goal of Level One is to build balanced strength in your abs and lower back. The number of repetitions you'll do in Level One is a little higher than the other levels. This will help build endurance in your muscles and help prevent injuries down the line. This base of strength and endurance is necessary for good posture. Good posture, which may sound old-fashioned, is essential for the health of your internal organs, good circulation, and increased energy flow. It also helps keep your lower back pain-free.

Pace

Depending on your fitness level, it is possible to reach the prescribed goals in three weeks, but everyone is different. If it takes you more time to fulfill these requirements, then that's the perfect pace for you. If you reach the goals in less time, then *hit the prescribed mark at least three times before you go to the next level*. These guidelines hold for all three levels.

Training Journal

At the end of each level, there will be a training-journal example. A training journal is a place to jot down thoughts, feelings, and insights about your workouts. Taking stock a few minutes after each workout or at the end of the week will keep your mind and body focused on your goals and on the process. This is different from a training log, which charts your progress in specific terms of exercise sets, reps, and so forth. The journal is more free-form and fluid. It is more like a workout diary. You may use the template at the end of each level as a model to create your own training journal.

The Workout Plan

There are several ways you can work the System into your schedule. You will need to work your abs four times a week and alternate between the Traditional Routine and the Functional Routine, doing each routine twice a week. I will give you three sample plans. Scheduling your workout time is not rocket science, but when you're in the middle of your own busy life, it's often difficult to get a clear perspective. These models will give you some ideas.

MIX IT UP/GO WITH THE FLOW

You can also mix it up. Each week may take on a life of its own. So you can switch things around. If the beginning of a week is just crazy and it is impossible to get in a workout on Monday, Tuesday, and Wednesday, you could do the program four straight days in a row (Thursday, Friday, Saturday, and Sunday).

SAMPLE PLAN ONE:

This plan sets your schedule during the week so your weekends are free.

- Monday: the Traditional Routine
- Tuesday: the Functional Routine
- Wednesday: rest day
- Thursday: the Traditional Routine
- Friday: the Functional Routine
- Saturday and Sunday: rest days

SAMPLE PLAN TWO:

This plan shifts two workout days to the weekend. If your workweek is incredibly hectic, this can be a better schedule.

- Monday: rest day
- Tuesday: the Traditional Routine
- Wednesday: the Functional Routine
- Thursday: rest day
- Friday: rest day
- Saturday: the Traditional Routine
- Sunday: the Functional Routine

SAMPLE PLAN THREE:

This plan is a compromise. It gives you one free day on the weekend, either Saturday or Sunday. This way, you'll have one day to just relax and not worry about work or working out. It's your day to do laundry, food shop, clean the bathroom, go to a movie.

- Monday: the Traditional Routine
- Tuesday: the Functional Routine
- Wednesday: rest day
- Thursday: the Traditional Routine
- Friday: rest day
- Saturday: the Functional Routine
- Sunday: rest day

Routine One:
The Traditional Routine

The Prescription: Work up to the prescribed repetitions and holds before moving on to the next level.

EXERCISE	REPETITIONS	SETS	PEAK HOLD
Reverse Crunches	20	1	2 seconds
Catches	10 on each side	1	2 seconds
Toe Touches	20	1	2 seconds
Basic Trunk Extensions	20	1	2 seconds

■ Reverse Crunches

DIFFICULTY: 2
LOWER BACK: LOW RISK
AREA OF FOCUS: LOWER ABS

STARTING POSITION: Lie flat on your back and raise your thighs so your knees are above your hips, placing your lower legs (calves and feet) parallel to the floor. You can place your hands either at your sides or behind your head. Refer to Both Hands Behind Head (page 18). (See photos on page 160.)

THE MOVE: Focusing on your lower abs, curl your hips off the floor toward your rib cage, moving your knees toward your forehead so your hips come off the ground two to three inches. Hold the contraction at the top of the movement. Then lower your hips in a controlled motion, keeping tension on your abs. As your hips touch the floor, repeat the movement.

TRAINER'S TIPS

- Make sure your abs are doing the work. Don't rock, using momentum.
- Don't rest your hips on the floor at the end of the movement.
- Keep constant tension on your abs.
- If your hands are at your sides, make sure you're using them just for balance and not to push off.
- Focus your mind on your lower abs.

■ Catches

DIFFICULTY: 1
LOWER BACK: LOW RISK
AREA OF FOCUS: OBLIQUES

STARTING POSITION: Lie flat on your back with your knees bent, both feet on the floor, and your arms extended toward your knees. (See photos on page 173.)

THE MOVE: Use your ab muscles to raise your torso diagonally, bringing your right shoulder across the centerline of your body and both hands outside and above your left knee, as if you were going to catch a ball. Hold the contraction at the top of the movement. Then, in a controlled motion, lower your torso back to the floor for one rep. Repeat the movement with your left shoulder.

TRAINER'S TIPS

- Make sure you get both arms outside your knee and slightly above knee level.
- Keep your lower back supported on the floor.
- Focus your mind on your oblique muscles.

■ Toe Touches

DIFFICULTY: 1
LOWER BACK: LOW RISK
AREA OF FOCUS: UPPER ABS

STARTING POSITION: Lie flat on your back with your legs straight up, perpendicular to your body (knees unlocked), and your arms extended straight up. (See photos on page 191.)

THE MOVE: Use your upper abs to raise your hands toward your toes. Hold the contraction at the top of the movement. Then, in a controlled motion, lower your torso back to the starting position, letting your shoulder blades lightly touch the floor. Repeat the movement.

TRAINER'S TIPS

- Don't rest at the bottom of the movement. When you feel your shoulder blades touch, start the next repetition.
- Don't worry about actually touching your toes. The objective is to get your shoulder blades off the ground two or three inches.
- Hold the peak contraction for the prescribed time.
- If you have problems holding your legs perpendicular, get them as close to the position as you can or hold them up against a wall.

■ Basic Trunk Extensions

DIFFICULTY: 1
LOWER BACK: LOW RISK
AREA OF FOCUS: LUMBAR EXTENSORS

STARTING POSITION: Lie on your stomach and rest your forehead on your hands. Your hands should be placed palms down on top of each other. (See photos on page 248.)

THE MOVE: Lengthening your spine, raise your torso and your head off the floor as high as you can while keeping your hips and feet in place. Hold the contraction at the top of the movement. Then, in a controlled motion, lower your body back to the starting position. Repeat the movement.

TRAINER'S TIPS

- Throughout the movement, think of lengthening your spine, so that the exercise is making you longer and taller.
- Keep your butt and leg muscles tight to protect your lower back.
- Focus on feeling and isolating your lower-back muscles as you raise your torso.

Routine Two: The Functional Routine

PEP TALK

This routine looks at your middle three-dimensionally and emphasizes your core. The exercises in this routine focus on multi-muscle movements.

It's important at this stage of your training to be patient. You're not going to see immediate results. Consistency is the key. Doing a little bit every day will add up. Just keep making deposits in your fitness bank account.

The Prescription: Work up to the prescribed repetitions and holds before moving on to the next level.

EXERCISE	REPETITIONS	SETS	PEAK HOLD
Swimming on Back	15 on each side	1	2 seconds
Swimming on Belly	15 on each side	1	2 seconds
Plank Series		1	30 seconds on each of four sides

■ Swimming on Back

DIFFICULTY: 2
LOWER BACK: MODERATE RISK
AREA OF FOCUS:
   ABDOMINAL MUSCLES

STARTING POSITION: Lie flat on your back with your legs fully extended on the floor and your arms extended over your head. (See photos on page 251.)

THE MOVE: Simultaneously raise your left arm and your right leg. Hold the contraction at the top of the movement. Lower your arm and leg until they lightly touch the floor. Repeat the movement with your right arm and left leg.

TRAINER'S TIPS

- Before you raise your arm and leg, extend your spine by lengthening the arm and leg you are going to raise.
- As you raise your arm, your shoulder blade will rise off the floor.
- Feel the movement initiating from the center of your body.
- Control both the up and the down phases of the movement.
- Keep your neck lengthened and in the proper position.

■ Swimming on Belly

DIFFICULTY: 2
LOWER BACK: MODERATE RISK
AREA OF FOCUS:
  LOWER-BACK MUSCLES

STARTING POSITION: Lie on your stomach with your legs fully extended on the floor and your arms extended over your head. Your head should be facing straight down. (See photos on page 252.)

THE MOVE: Simultaneously raise your left arm and your right leg. Hold the contraction at the top of the movement. Lower your arm and leg until they lightly touch the floor. Repeat the movement with your right arm and left leg.

TRAINER'S TIPS

- Before you raise your arm and leg, extend your spine by lengthening the arm and leg you are going to raise.
- Feel the movement initiating from the center of your body.
- Control both the up and the down phases of the movement.
- Hold the peak contraction for the prescribed time.
- Keep your neck lengthened.

■ Plank Series

DIFFICULTY: 2
LOWER BACK: LOW RISK
AREA OF FOCUS: CORE

POSITION ONE: DOWN PLANK: Lie on your stomach; raise your body off the floor and support yourself on your forearms (or hands) and your toes. Raise your hips so your body is as straight as a board. Hold for the prescribed time. (See photos on page 257.)

POSITION TWO: SIDE PLANK: Lie on your left side; rest on your left forearm (or hand) and the outside edge of your left foot. Raise your hips so your body is as straight as a board. Hold for the prescribed time.

POSITION THREE: SIDE PLANK: Lie on your right side; rest on your right forearm (or hand) and the outside edge of your right foot. Raise your hips so your body is as straight as a board. Hold for the prescribed time.

POSITION FOUR: UP PLANK: Lie on your back; rest on your forearms (or hands) and your heels. Raise your hips so your body is as straight as a board. Hold for the prescribed time.

TRAINER'S TIPS

- Focus on keeping your body as straight as a board.
- Don't let your hips sag.
- Keep your neck lengthened and in line with your spine. This will also work your neck-stabilization muscles.

Training Journal: A Sampling of Entries

The following are examples of thoughts you might record in a journal. Each thought could be expanded or serve as a simple reminder, like on a to-do list.

- Focus on technique during each exercise.
- I need to be patient. I'm not going to perfect each movement right off the bat.
- When I'm crunching and I'm getting tired, I noticed I bring my head forward instead of keeping proper spacing.
- On reverse crunches, I kick my lower legs up to help my hips off the floor. Keep it strict.
- Don't expect results overnight, no miracles like in the television commercials. I have to stay with it.
- This isn't so bad. I can stay with this.
- After just doing the first level, I'm starting to get back in touch with my body. So many things just feel like habits. I sit in a chair all day at work, then I come home and lounge on the couch. But I have a choice. I can create my own habits. When I work out, I have more energy. It opens up new choices.
- As a reward, when I finish Level One, I'm going to treat myself to dinner at my favorite restaurant.

CHAPTER FOUR

The System: Level Two

REQUIRED READING:
CHAPTER SEVEN, "THE MIND"

Pep Talk

Congratulations, you've made it to Level Two. Now that you're feeling a little more comfortable with the process, it's time to take your exercise awareness to the next level, especially with the movements you learned in Level One. Try to perform each exercise with precision, and focus your mind on the working muscle(s).

The purpose of this level is twofold: to get you over the hump of creating a new habit and to increase the endurance of your ab muscles.

A warning: The middle is a dangerous place. It's too early to see any results, and the excitement of getting started has faded. Focus on the health benefits—on how you feel, not how you look. You need to know that a healthy lifestyle is not vain and selfish. It is giving. It gives you more energy and can give you a longer and more productive life, so you can give more to those you love and to the world.

Goals

Here's the upside: By adding new exercises, this level will increase the strength and endurance in your abs and lower back. As your posture continues to improve, your energy levels will increase. By the end of this level, you will notice that your center is firmer and stronger.

Routine One: The Traditional Routine

The Prescription: Work up to the prescribed repetitions and holds before moving on to the next level.

EXERCISE	REPETITIONS	SETS	PEAK HOLD
Hip-Ups	15	1	2 seconds
Reverse Crunches	15	1	2 seconds
Crossovers	15 on each side	1	2 seconds
Catches	15 on each side	1	2 seconds
Butterfly Crunches	15	1	2 seconds
Toe Touches	15	1	2 seconds
Intermediate Trunk Extensions	15	1	2 seconds

■ Hip-Ups

DIFFICULTY: 2
LOWER BACK: MODERATE RISK
AREA OF FOCUS: LOWER ABS

STARTING POSITION: Lie flat on your back with your legs straight up, perpendicular to your body (knees unlocked). Place your hands at your sides, palms down, and keep your neck long and your head aligned with your spine. (See photos on page 161.)

THE MOVE: Use your lower abs to raise your hips off the floor, bringing your hips slightly toward your rib cage. Hold the contraction at the top of the movement. Lower your hips back to the starting position until they lightly touch the floor. Repeat the movement.

TRAINER'S TIPS

- Don't kick up with your legs or push off with your hands to get your hips up—use your ab muscles.
- Hold the peak contraction for the prescribed time.
- Control both the up and the down phases of the movement.
- Focus your mind on your lower abs.

■ Reverse Crunches *(page 32)*

■ Crossovers

DIFFICULTY: 2
LOWER BACK: MODERATE RISK
AREA OF FOCUS: OBLIQUES

STARTING POSITION: Lie flat on your back with your knees bent and both feet on the floor. Then cross your left ankle over your right knee, making a triangle between your legs. Your right hand goes behind your head, elbow extended. Your left hand can either rest extended at your left side or, preferably, rest on your right side, so you can feel your obliques work. (See photos on page 172.)

THE MOVE: Use your abs to raise and cross your right shoulder toward your left knee. Hold the contraction at the top of the movement. Lower your body back to the starting position until your shoulder blades lightly touch the floor. Repeat on the other side.

TRAINER'S TIPS

- Make sure your torso twists toward your knee. Don't just reach with your elbow.
- Make sure you are also raising your torso up, not just rolling it to the left.
- Control both the up and the down phases of the movement.
- Hold the peak contraction for the prescribed time.
- Focus your mind on your obliques.

■ Catches *(page 32)*

■ Butterfly Crunches

DIFFICULTY: 1
LOWER BACK: LOW RISK
AREA OF FOCUS: UPPER ABS

STARTING POSITION: Lying flat on your back, bring the soles of your feet together and let your knees fall to the sides. Put your hands in the position of choice. (See photos on page 190.)

THE MOVE: Raise your shoulder blades off the floor two to three inches by curling your rib cage toward your hips. Hold the contraction at the top of the movement. Then lower your shoulder blades back to the starting position. Repeat the movement.

TRAINER'S TIPS

- Keep your spine neutral.
- Keep constant tension on your ab muscles, controlling both the up and the down phases of the movement.
- Hold the peak contraction for the prescribed time.
- Keep the proper positioning between your chin and chest.

■ Toe Touches *(page 33)*

■ Intermediate Trunk Extensions

DIFFICULTY: 2
LOWER BACK: MODERATE RISK
AREA OF FOCUS: LUMBAR EXTENSORS

STARTING POSITION: Lay a firm cushion under your hips as you lie on your stomach. Then rest your forehead on your hands. Your hands should be placed palms down on top of each other.

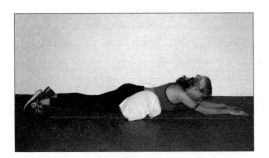

THE MOVE: Lengthening your spine, raise your torso and your head off the floor as high as you can, keeping your head aligned with your spine as you move and keeping your feet in place. Hold the contraction at the top of the movement. Lower your body back to the starting position. Repeat the movement.

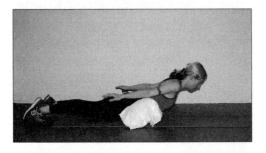

TRAINER'S TIPS

- The pillow under your hips increases your range of motion. The bigger and bulkier the object, the larger the range of motion. So a rolled-up towel would be easier than a firm pillow or two towels rolled up.
- Gradually increase the size of the object under your hips as you feel more comfortable.
- Throughout the movement, think of lengthening the spine, so the exercise is making you longer and taller.
- Keep your butt and leg muscles tight to protect your lower back.
- Focus on feeling and isolating your lower-back muscles as you raise your torso.
- You can also use a workout ball.

Routine Two:
The Functional Routine

You have probably experienced the feeling of not wanting to work out, of not feeling motivated, and of not being able to do what you did the last workout. These setbacks aren't what they appear to be. A setback is often preparation for a couple of leaps forward. Persevering through these tough days is part of the journey to the next level. So stick with it and believe in the great leap forward.

The Prescription: Work up to the prescribed repetitions and holds before moving on to the next level.

EXERCISE	REPETITIONS	SETS	PEAK HOLD
Swimming on Back	15 on each side	1	2 seconds
Swimming on Belly	15 on each side	1	2 seconds
Reverse Superwomans	15	1	2 seconds
Superwomans	20	1	2 seconds
Plank Series		1	45 seconds on each of four sides
Vacuum Pumps	15	1	2 seconds

■ Swimming on Back
(page 34)

■ Swimming on Belly *(page 35)*

■ Reverse Superwomans

DIFFICULTY: 2
LOWER BACK: MODERATE RISK
AREA OF FOCUS:
   ABDOMINAL MUSCLES

STARTING POSITION: Lie flat on your back with your legs fully extended on the floor and your arms extended over your head. (See photos on page 254.)

THE MOVE: Simultaneously raise your arms, shoulder blades, and legs off the floor. Hold the contraction at the top of the movement. Lower your arms, shoulder blades, and legs until they lightly touch the floor. Repeat the movement.

TRAINER'S TIPS

- Before you raise your arms and legs, lengthen your spine by stretching your arms and legs in opposite directions, as if they were being pulled.
- Feel the movement initiating from the center of your body.
- Control both the up and the down phases of the movement.

■ Superwomans

DIFFICULTY: 2
LOWER BACK: MODERATE RISK
AREA OF FOCUS:
LOWER-BACK MUSCLES

STARTING POSITION: Lie on your stomach with your legs fully extended on the floor and your arms extended over your head. Your head should be facing straight down. (See photos on page 253.)

THE MOVE: Simultaneously raise your arms, torso, and legs, as if your were flying. Hold the contraction at the top of the movement. Lower your arms, torso, and legs until they lightly touch the floor. Repeat the movement.

TRAINER'S TIPS

- Before you raise your arms and legs, lengthen your spine by stretching your arms and legs in opposite directions, as if they were being pulled.
- Feel the movement initiating from the center of your body.
- Control both the up and the down phases of the movement.
- Hold the peak contraction for the prescribed time.

■ Plank Series *(page 35)*

■ Vacuum Pumps

DIFFICULTY: 2
LOWER BACK: LOW RISK
AREA OF FOCUS:
TRANSVERSE ABDOMINIS

STARTING POSITIONS: (1) On all fours. (2) Kneeling, hands on thighs, heels on buttocks, and back straight. (3) Standing, legs slightly bent and hands on thighs. (See photos on page 225.)

THE MOVE: Exhale all the air from your body and suck your abdomen up and in as far as you can. Hold for 10 seconds. Relax and repeat.

TRAINER'S TIPS

- Focus your mind on pulling your abs up and in.
- Each starting position will get progressively harder, all fours being the easiest and standing the hardest.
- Start out holding each exhalation for 10 seconds and gradually work up to 30 seconds.

Training Journal:
A Sampling of Entries

- Make sure I review proper techniques for new exercises.
- I need to push myself a little harder each workout.
- Focus on the process, not results.
- When I don't feel like working out but I do it anyway, I feel so much better.
- Visualize my perfect abs at night before I go to sleep.
- I need to keep my rest time down between exercises.
- As a reward for finishing Level Two, I'm going to treat myself to an hour massage.
- At times, I struggled to get through these three weeks. But now I feel like I've really made it to a new place. I'm excited about Level Three. I know there will be challenges, but now there is no turning back.

CHAPTER FIVE

The System: Level Three

REQUIRED READING:
CHAPTER EIGHT, "KNOW YOURSELF"

Pep Talk

Congratulations, you've made it to Level Three. Keep challenging yourself to bring your mind and your body together during your workouts. If you've ever taken a yoga class, you know how important it is to stay present in the room and focus on the posture. You need to bring the same focus to these workouts. Yoga does not have a corner on the market with the mind-body principle. Connect your mind to the area you are working and stay focused on each repetition. Don't think about the office. Don't think about what movie you want to rent. Don't think about what to wear to dinner. Focus in the moment, and when you're finished, your mind will be refreshed and ready to solve any problem.

This level asks more of you. Face the challenge in the spirit of fun. The good news is that by the time you complete this level, you will be able to see a difference.

This level adds three new intense exercises. If these exercises are too difficult or feel dangerous for your lower back, repeat the Level Two exercise for that ab area. For example, if you can't perform corkscrews, do two sets of hip-ups for the recommended repetitions.

durance, and working out will be integrated into your lifestyle. That's big!

Start to use the visualization techniques you've learned. Be able to see the body you want. See a snapshot of that image before you work out and when you're done.

Goals

Here's the upside in completing these next three weeks: Your level of concentration will increase as your workout time increases, your abs and lower back will reach an even higher level of strength and en-

Routine One: The Traditional Routine

The Prescription: Work up to the prescribed repetitions and holds before moving on to the next level.

EXERCISE	REPETITIONS	SETS	PEAK HOLD
Corkscrews	8 on each side	1	2 seconds
Hip-Ups	15	1	2 seconds
Reverse Crunches	15	1	2 seconds
Bent-Knee Leg-Overs	15 on each side	1	2 seconds
Catches	15 on each side	1	2 seconds
Crossovers	15 on each side	1	2 seconds
Crunches	15	1	2 seconds
Butterfly Crunches	15	1	2 seconds
Toe Touches	15	1	2 seconds
Intermediate Trunk Extensions	15	1	2 seconds
Trunk Extensions with Rotation	15	1	2 seconds

■ Corkscrews

DIFFICULTY: 3
LOWER BACK: HIGH RISK
AREA OF FOCUS: LOWER ABS AND
**   LOWER OBLIQUES**

STARTING POSITION: Lie flat on your back with your legs straight up, perpendicular to your body (knees unlocked). Place your hands at your sides, palms down, for support. (See photos on page 162.)

THE MOVE: Raise and twist your hips off the floor in a corkscrew motion to the left. Hold the contraction at the top of the movement. Lower your hips back to the starting position until they lightly touch the floor. Repeat the movement, twisting your hips to the right.

TRAINER'S TIPS

- Don't rest at the bottom of the movement.
- Control both the up and the down phases of the movement.
- Hold the peak contraction for the prescribed time.
- Don't kick your legs up. Use your abs to elevate them.
- Use your hands for stability, not to push off.
- Focus on your lower abs and lower obliques.
- Keep your legs perpendicular throughout the exercise. Don't lower them back to the ground.
- Keep your neck lengthened.

■ Hip-Ups *(page 38)*

■ Reverse Crunches *(page 32)*

■ Bent-Knee Leg-Overs

DIFFICULTY: 2
LOWER BACK: LOW RISK
AREA OF FOCUS: OBLIQUES

STARTING POSITION: Lie flat on your back with your hands spread out perpendicular to your body. Raise your knees directly above your hips with your lower legs extended parallel to the floor. (See photos on page 182.)

THE MOVE: Use your oblique muscles to lower both knees to your right side, so the outside of your right thigh gently touches the floor. Hold the contraction at the top of the movement. Raise your knees back to the starting position. Repeat the movement, lowering your knees to your left side.

TRAINER'S TIPS

- As you lower your legs to the side, let your hips roll in the same direction.
- Try to keep both shoulder blades on the floor throughout the movement.
- Focus on feeling your obliques do the work.
- Keep your neck lengthened.

■ **Catches** *(page 32)*

■ **Crossovers** *(page 39)*

■ **Crunches**

DIFFICULTY: 1
LOWER BACK: LOW RISK
AREA OF FOCUS: UPPER ABS

STARTING POSITION: Lie flat on your back with your knees bent and both feet on the floor, your hands in the position of choice. (See photos on page 188.)

THE MOVE: Raise and curl your shoulder blades off the floor. Hold the contraction at the top of the movement. Lower your upper body back to the starting position, letting your shoulder blades lightly touch the floor. Repeat the movement.

TRAINER'S TIPS

- Keep tension on your abs throughout the movement.
- Don't rest at the bottom of the movement.
- Hold the peak contraction for the prescribed time.
- Make sure your shoulder blades come off the floor. Don't move just your head up and down.
- Keep the small of your back against the floor.
- Focus on your upper abs.

■ **Butterfly Crunches** *(page 39)*

■ **Toe Touches** *(page 33)*

■ **Intermediate Trunk Extensions** *(page 40)*

■ **Trunk Extensions with Rotation**

DIFFICULTY: 2
LOWER BACK: MODERATE RISK
AREA OF FOCUS: LUMBAR EXTENSORS

STARTING POSITION: Lie on your stomach and rest your forehead on your hands. Your hands should be placed one on top of the other. (See photos on page 249.)

THE MOVE: Lengthening your spine, raise your torso off the floor and rotate your right shoulder up as you turn your head in the same direction. Hold the contraction at the top of the movement. Lower your torso back to the starting position. Repeat the movement, rotating up and to your left.

TRAINER'S TIPS

- Throughout the movement, think of lengthening your spine, so the exercise is making you longer and taller.
- Keep your butt and leg muscles tight to protect your lower back.
- Focus on feeling and isolating your lower-back muscles as you raise and turn your torso.
- Keep your neck lengthened.

Routine Two: The Functional Routine

PEP TALK

Consistency of effort is the key. You will *not* always have consistency with your results. Life will continue to create stressful obstacles: work, relationships, family. Some nights, you're just not going to get much sleep and this will affect your workout. But you can give each workout a solid effort. In fact, that's all you can do. Even if the workouts seem like drudgery, they are actually releasing stress and combating anxiety, and in the long run, they will help you sleep better.

As you approach these last three weeks, it is important to start adding other fitness elements to your program (if you haven't already). This week, start with the cardio program (page 99). Next week, add the weight-training program (page 100) and the stretching routine (page 96). The programs in this book will ease you into these routines gradually, so don't be intimidated.

The Prescription: Work up to the prescribed repetitions and holds before moving on to the next level.

EXERCISE	REPETITIONS	SETS	PEAK HOLD
Swimming on Back	20 on each side	1	2 seconds
Swimming on Belly	20 on each side	1	2 seconds
Reverse Superwomans	20	1	2 seconds
Superwomans	20	1	2 seconds
Side Superwomans	20 on each side	1	2 seconds
Plank Series		1	45 seconds on each of four sides
Vacuum Pumps	15	1	2 seconds

■ **Swimming on Back** *(page 34)*

■ **Swimming on Belly** *(page 35)*

■ **Reverse Superwomans** *(page 41)*

■ **Superwomans** *(page 42)*

■ Side Superwomans

DIFFICULTY: 3
LOWER BACK: MODERATE RISK
AREA OF FOCUS: OBLIQUES AND
STABILIZATION MUSCLES

STARTING POSITION: Lie on your left side with your legs and arms fully extended. (See photos on page 256.)

THE MOVE: Simultaneously raise your arms, torso, and legs, as if your were flying on your side. Hold the contraction at the top of the movement. Lower your arms and legs until they lightly touch the floor. Repeat the movement until you have completed your set. Then switch sides.

TRAINER'S TIPS

- Before you raise your arms and legs, lengthen your spine by stretching your arms and legs in opposite directions, as if they were being pulled.
- Feel the movement initiating from the center of your body.
- Try to keep your elbows in line with your ears.
- Control both the up and the down phases of the movement.
- Hold the peak contraction for the prescribed time.

■ Plank Series *(page 35)*

■ Vacuum Pumps *(page 42)*

Training Journal: A Sampling of Entries

- Take pride in my technique, like it's a dance.
- I need to push myself a little harder each workout. Keep raising my intensity.
- Visualize my perfect abs at night before I go to sleep.
- Stay focused rep by rep. Quality.
- This is my time for myself. A time-out from the daily grind.
- As a reward for finishing Level Three, I'm going to treat myself to an afternoon at a spa.
- It feels so good to complete the program. I'm excited about making progress with the weights, running, and stretching. It's amazing that it doesn't take that long to do all these things. And I have so much more energy. I feel like I've got my body back— not just my body, a little sanity, too.

The Next Step

Congratulations, you've finished the core program. Now what? Usually when a team wins a championship, they immediately start to talk about the repeat. You need to think about your next step, your new exercise goals. This isn't brain science. You need to be honest and realistic. Stay on the program in a way that fits your lifestyle. The following suggestions will give you some ideas for taking it to the next level.

- Push your aerobic workout up to thirty-five or forty minutes and do it four times a week.
- Add weight resistance to your ab program.
- Remember, the body works in cycles. Keep switching your routine.
- Increase the intensity of your weight-training program.
- Hire a personal trainer for a month. Then do it on your own again.

These choices should take care of your ab training for years to come. You can also treat yourself to another fitness book for inspiration.

THE COMPLETE EXERCISER

As you take off on your journey, keep the following steps in mind.

Step One: Knowledge. You need to know what you're doing. When it comes to your abs, this means doing the exercises properly and following the routines.

Step Two: Discipline. You need to train with consistency. You have to put your knowledge into action for the long term.

Step Three: Motivation. You need to find deep ways to stay motivated, or else you'll struggle to stay consistent.

Step Four: Letting Go. Release the need for control and results. Focus on the process. This is a paradox. You need to plan, dream, and work hard, while at the same time, you need to roll with the punches. As T. S. Eliot said, "The secret is to care and not to care. The caring is in the preparation. The not caring is in the letting go."

As the old saying goes, "Train hard. Train Smart. Train with consistency. Have fun."

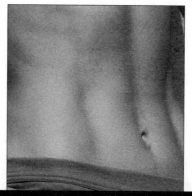

PART THREE

The Reader

The Reader supplements the nuts-and-bolts information of Part One, "The Foundation." This section will introduce you to basic concepts of lower-back care, exercise physiology for women, and nutrition. It will also cover important mental skills such as setting goals, getting motivated, visualizing, and staying focused in the moment. These assignments can be read interactively with Part Two, "The System," or they can be read as self-contained chapters.

CHAPTER SIX

Reader One: The Body

Assignment #1: Lower-Back Basics

PREVIEW: *This section explains the importance of training your lower back and analyzes how lower-back problems develop.*

THE PROBLEM

As a culture, we overtrain the front of our bodies—especially our abs. This is what we look at in the mirror and what we present to the world. The lower back never makes the glossy covers of national magazines, so we hardly spend any time training or thinking about it. Because we neglect the lower back, the muscles weaken, which can lead to chronic lower-back pain. We might train our lower backs with more zeal if we could look forward to getting compliments like, "Wow, you have a really sexy lower back." Since this isn't likely to happen, it's important to understand why you need to train your lower back. This section will explain lower-back basics. To know the good is to do the good. And a strong lower back, I daresay, is a sexy lower back.

BIOMECHANICS

The main group of lower back muscles you need to be concerned about are the erector spinae. These muscles are extensors. They help you extend and straighten your torso. As the name implies, they also help keep you erect. They help stabilize your torso and assist in twisting movements, as well.

These muscles are like steel cables that support and secure the spine. They run up and down the spine, attaching to the ribs, the hips, and other areas of support to secure and protect the spine. Like the masterful muscle design of the abs, the spinal erectors work with smaller inner muscles, like the multifidus, to secure individual vertebrae. These muscles create an architecture for support and movement.

The Buddy System

The abdominal and lower-back muscles are partners. They have opposite functions, yet they complement each other, working together like a team. What would life be like without them? If the erector spinae didn't exist, your torso would drop forward and you wouldn't be able to raise yourself up. If you didn't have your ab muscles, your torso would fall over backward and you wouldn't be able to pull yourself up and forward. Together they are in a constant dance of balance, a beautiful tension of opposites, keeping you upright and functional. If your abs are weak, it puts an extra load on your lower back, disks, and vertebrae. If your lower back is weak, it puts an extra load on your abs. An imbalance creates structural problems. That's why you must train your lower back and your abs.

HOW LOWER BACK PAIN DEVELOPS

The Unguarded Moment. Back pain can begin obviously with a traumatic event, such as an accident. Or it can happen, as it often does, in an unguarded moment—when you step off a curb, twist to pick up a bag of groceries, or even sneeze. If your lower back is unable to withstand the force of these movements, then you feel that little tweak or that sharp or shooting pain.

The Spiral from Acute to Chronic. Once you have suffered an injury, you start to protect the injured area. This, of course, is a natural and healthy response. This guards the injured muscle from external forces that could do more damage, and helps relieve short-term pain. Over time, however, this guarding weakens the muscle through disuse. As muscles get weaker and weaker, they become more prone to injury. A weak muscle is a vulnerable muscle. The weaker it becomes, the less it takes to injure it. Soon it can't even withstand daily activities, and you are in constant pain.

The Weak Link. The main problem is what I mentioned earlier: The lower back is the area we most often neglect to train because it's not a sexual hot spot like the abs, butt, or chest. Since it is neglected, it is the area most likely to fall into this cycle. That's why back pain and injury are such major health issues.

Training the Weak Link. The good news is, you can train this area, bringing your body back into balance. Strengthening these muscles through consistent exercise is one of the best ways to prevent and rehabilitate lower-back problems.

TRAINING YOUR LOWER BACK

The System is designed to train your torso—front, back, and sides. You need to train your lower back to keep it strong. Here are some guidelines:

• Always work your lower-back muscles within a comfortable range of motion where you feel no pain.
• Stop movement just prior to the point of discomfort. You will receive strength benefits beyond the range of motion. This will always give you a safe buffer of strength.
• Don't use sudden movements.
• Perform movements in a slow and controlled manner.

To Sum Up

The above guidelines illustrate an important point when it comes to training your lower back: Be careful. Since this is a vulnerable area, the chances of injury increase. So heed the advice—stop the movement just prior to discomfort. You will still receive strength benefits. Build a solid foundation; then you can start to push it a little. These aren't muscles you want to shock. They are muscles you want to coax, to invite in a friendly way. Give yourself at least three months of consistent work before you start to push it. The Lower-Back Routine, found in Part Six (page 147), is perfect for building this foundation.

Assignment #2: An Exercise Primer for Women

PREVIEW: *This section covers a short list of the things you should know about your body, from body image to hormones. We will look at how exercise and our culture at large affect the way you use and see your body.*

OUR CULTURE

You may be asking, what can a man know about female body image? Actually, there are a couple of reasons why I can relate. The first is my experience as a personal trainer. Every female client I've worked with—whether she was a model, an actress, or a businesswoman—believed she was overweight. In 90 percent of these cases, the women were not overweight. Even after they trained and lost weight, they still thought they were overweight. It made me believe in the popular maxim: "A woman can never be too thin and a man can never be too rich." They all wanted the perfect body. The perfect body, of course, is unattainable.

Whenever I give a seminar on ab training, I like to start with a little free association. I'll ask the class what words come to mind when I say "abs." It always goes something like this: *ripped, shredded, defined, six-pack, gut, blob, jelly-belly, pooch, pudding.* It is either perfection or failure, no happy medium. Either you're one of the lucky ones or an ab-loser.

This says a lot about the way our culture sees the body, especially the abs. It's a world of haves and have-nots. Either we have that six-pack or we're chubby. It is nearly impossible to feel any other way, because we are constantly bombarded by images of perfection. Our minds are tattooed with flawless pictures from billboards, magazines, TV, and movies. These images represent the perfect body—superslim, toned, airbrushed, and transformed by the miracles of plastic surgery. It is surreal and disorienting to see celebrities in their early sixties now looking like they are in their twenties, their faces Botoxed and pulled unnaturally tight and smooth.

Okay, now I feel like I need to confess. The second reason I can relate is that I *am* a man. I, too, constantly feel like I need to be working harder to measure up. Should I get a chemical peel? Am I a failure if I'm not ripped like the guy in the underwear advertisement? I, too, hear that body-image voice in my head chastising me, taunting me.

Nowadays men also feel the need to be perfect—like they have to have an abdominal six-pack and a full head of hair and look ten years younger than their age. With the recent trend of implants, men are now putting their health on the line to measure up, just like women. I'm not saying men have it as bad as women. We don't. The pressure that women have to attain the perfect body is still far greater than what our culture places on men. But I can understand on a personal level, too.

THE CONSTRUCTION OF BEAUTY

As long as I'm confessing—I used to be a body-part model, primarily for abs. My claim to fame is that I once modeled a jockstrap for a medical catalog. Besides working very hard to stay in great shape, I had to learn all the tricks: Every time the camera clicks, the model is flexing the ab muscles hard and tight and expelling all the air from his or her body. This is not a functional, moving, and breathing body. It is a poser body, a kind of imposter, a chameleon who changes form for the camera. The images of beauty that we aspire to are not real. They are constructed.

Okay, so we have the posing model who has been dieting hard and is now flexing hard, then there's the expert lighting that highlights the strong points and hides the flaws in soft shadows. Technology has taken it a step farther. Through the techniques of airbrushing, augmenting, and compositing, magazine covers now feature virtual women. The nose is touched up, the lips are made fuller, and body parts are actually taken from other images. A famous example of this was the movie poster for *Pretty Woman,* featuring Richard Gere and Julia Roberts. They used Julia Roberts's face but not her body. She didn't make the cut. Even real-life sex symbols aren't good enough.

BODY IMAGE

In her documentary *Slim Hopes,* Jean Kilbourne, a leading body-image educator, quotes two studies. The first was targeted at women between the ages of thirty and fifty. They were asked what they would most want to change about their lives. The number one answer was to lose weight. The second study targeted girls between the ages of eleven and seventeen. The number one answer in this age group was to lose weight and keep it off.

Kilbourne believes the saddest thing about these results is the impoverishment of the imagination. This is where the mind dwells—instead of on careers, education, and the arts. Kilbourne says, "The obsession with body image and thinness cuts right to the heart of a woman's power, energy, and self-esteem."

So we see these constructed images, and then we see our own very real bodies in the mirror without all the magic of airbrushing and lighting. When we go to the beach, it is primarily the superfit who have the courage to wear the skimpy outfits. When Kathy Bates disrobed to get in a hot tub with Jack Nicholson in *About Schmidt,* it was a national story. I wish I was kidding, but it's the literal truth. It made all the talk shows and magazines. A woman who *isn't* lean and trim dared to disrobe. Stop the presses! An act unprecedented in mainstream American culture has occurred!

For most of us, it's been a long while since we've seen our peers naked without "lights, camera, action!" It might have been in junior high PE class or occasionally a close friend. At the health club, people tend to cover and run. It is difficult even in these socially acceptable situations. We still cover ourselves, not wanting to be judged.

The first step to health and wellness is to understand the facts, to become more conscious of the cultural pressures. Action is also needed. By action, I mean training your body and owning it with pride. These two things go hand in hand. And they are two crucial steps in empowering yourself.

VOCABULARY

Hemoglobin: A complex combination of protein and iron in red blood cells that transports oxygen to the muscles.

Adipose Tissue: A type of connective tissue containing fat cells that forms a layer under the skin. It serves as insulation, protection, and an energy reserve.

EXERCISE PHYSIOLOGY

Hormones: Testosterone and Estrogen

Your sex hormones are major players when it comes to body composition and exercise. As we talk about these two hormones, keep in mind that you have both testosterone and estrogen. As a woman, you have a higher percentage of estrogen. This hormone kicks in during puberty. Let's take a look at these powerful hormones.

Testosterone

Testosterone is found in greater quantities in the male body. In terms of body composition and exercise, testosterone has the following major effects:

- It builds muscle.
- It stimulates hemoglobin production, which increases the body's capacity to carry oxygen through the bloodstream.
- It decreases the amount of adipose tissue.

Estrogen

Estrogen is found in greater quantities in the female body. It is a more complex hormone. Natalie Angier, in her book *Woman: An Intimate Geography,* talks about the contradictions women must juggle when it comes to estrogen. Women are given the message that it is the hormone of the weaker sex and somehow inferior. Then, after menopause, women are told how important it is for a healthy heart, strong bones, and a clear mind. Angier summarizes the history of estrogen:

Over the years It [estrogen] has been demonized, glorified, excommunicated, and resurrected. . . . To appreciate estrogen, we need to begin by separating estrogen—what we know and don't know about its powers and constraints—from estrogen the parable, the imagined ingredient in Wicca's medicine chest, source of lunacy and the malign feminine.

As far as its powers, there are some perks to having estrogen as it relates to exercise. Colette Dowling, in her book *The Frailty Myth: Women Approaching Physical Equality*, cites recent studies that suggest two important benefits of estrogen.

• It buffers against muscle soreness after exercise.
• It allows women to endure longer exercise sessions.

The mix of estrogen and testosterone in your body makes a great partnership when it comes to working out.

The Body by Design

Men and women are designed to store different percentages of body fat. On average, women carry 18 to 26 percent of their body weight in fat. Men carry between 12 and 18 percent of their body weight in fat. This is the evolutionary design of nature.

The main reason for the higher fat percentage in women is the hormone estrogen. During puberty, estrogen changes the female body—hips widen, breasts develop, and menstruation begins. Estrogen increases the development of adipose tissue, which creates a container or a home for fat.

This adipose tissue forms the female pattern of fat storage. The normal areas of storage for women are the buttocks, abdominal area, hips, breasts, and thighs. The main reason for extra fat storage is to prepare for childbirth. It is natural that women store fat to protect certain areas and have a system to stockpile energy to nourish another person.

As a woman, it is difficult to get that hard, cut look like a man. This doesn't mean you have to go to drastic measures to get defined and toned muscles, but it will be extremely difficult and potentially unhealthy for you to pursue the same ripped six-pack as a man. Your body has its own aesthetic shape and this isn't the mirror image of the male physique. But remember, your body also contains testosterone, and adipose tissue does not hinder the development of lean body mass. A complete fitness program will systematically lower your body fat.

Too Lean

It is possible to be too lean. For a woman, going below 8 percent body fat can be a threat to health. You need a certain percentage of fat to protect your organs and to ensure proper nutrition. Extreme leanness has been linked to reproductive, circulatory, and immune system disorders. It can also be a sign of dangerous eating disorders, such as anorexia nervosa and bulimia nervosa.

Body Balance

It is important to stress again that your body naturally stores fat in the buttocks, abdominal area, hips, breasts, and thighs. When your fat falls within the normal percentages, this gives your body an attractive shape. It is only when you fall out of balance and gain excess weight that these natural aesthetic areas evolve into trouble spots. Most men adore the natural female shape and are turned off by the extremes, just as most women are not attracted to bodybuilders with huge overdeveloped muscles.

So, the goal is not to rid your body of the natural areas where you store fat, as the media and advertising images suggest, but to bring your body into an aesthetically pleasing and healthy balance.

Know Thyself

Differences at a Glance

According to the Mayo Clinic Women's Health Source, here are some of the differences between men's and women's bodies.

- Women have on average 11 percent more body fat and 8 percent less muscle mass than men.
- Men tend to be faster than women during aerobic events because of greater muscle strength.
- Women tend to have greater endurance capacity because of stored-fat energy.

Common Myths

Myth: Men are born stronger.

Fact: We are all born equal, but we develop differently and are socialized differently. The main physical differences don't happen at birth. They happen at puberty when the hormones kick in.

Myth: Boys are more coordinated than girls.

Fact: As far as developmental and motor-skill capabilities are concerned, there is no difference. Girls are just as coordinated as boys. Boys are encouraged to develop these skills, so there will be a difference in how skills evolve. If a girl plays sports from childhood through college, if she has a variety of physical pursuits—gymnastics, karate, dance, soccer, and basketball—her physical skills will reach a high level. If a boy sits in front of the computer screen all day and eats fast food day in and day out, then his physical skills will be dwarfed by his female counterpart. He'll get his butt kicked in karate, on the court, and on the field. What if this was the norm for our culture?

Myth: Men have better muscles.

Fact: This is not true. Men have more muscle, but it's a matter of quantity, not quality. If scientists looked through a microscope at a man's muscle tissue and a woman's muscle tissue, they couldn't say, "Oh, this is the man's muscle tissue and this is the woman's."

The Great Equalizer

Exercise is the great equalizer. The difference between men and women is not about *quality* but about *quantity*. Men have more muscle and store less fat. You can increase your lean body mass by working out and being active. Closing this gap is not about trying to look like a ripped man. That goes against how your body works. The goal is to achieve a healthy, functional, and aesthetically pleasing body.

To do this, you have to let go of the unhealthy myths and the other obstacles that our culture tries to impose on what it means to be a woman. These myths and obstacles create perpetual dissatisfaction with your body. This is unhealthy for your mind and body. Your body wants to look and *be* strong, healthy, toned, and vibrant. Starting on a workout program is an important step in empowering your body.

Assignment #3: Nutrition

PREVIEW: *This section goes back to the basics of nutrition to look at why we eat and outlines some commonsense principles for a healthy eating.*

A DANGEROUS CONVERSATION

Eating has become a controversial subject. It could go on the list with politics and religion as topics not to discuss with friends and family. One minute, you're having a civil conversation about diet, and the next thing you know, it's a holy war. It's the truth according to Atkins versus the truth according to Dean Ornish; then Barry Sears shows up and he's in the Zone and it's a wrestling death match. Then a vegetarian comes through the door and all hell breaks loose.

There are so many diet books and experts who spend their whole lives researching, testing, fighting, and disagreeing that it seems impossible to untangle the truth or give advice that would work for most readers. Do you feel as overwhelmed and confused as I do?

In this section, we're going to go old-school and talk about eating basics, giving you a solid foundation of knowledge. These basics will help you analyze diets and food choices.

THE BASICS

Why Do We Eat?

The first question, although obvious, is not often asked: Why do we eat? There are three main reasons—to give the body energy, to repair and rebuild, and to give the body the essential vitamins and minerals it needs. So a diet should fulfill these needs in an efficient and natural way. As basic as this question is, it is something you probably don't ask when you make food choices or go on a diet.

The goal is never to have to use the word *diet*. If you eat a variety of healthy foods in the proper proportion, and if you exercise and stay active, weight will not be an issue, and the whole concept of dieting will be obsolete.

Calories: The Basic Unit

Energy from food is measured in the form of calories. Our calories come from three primary sources: fats, carbohydrates, and proteins. These sources contain calories in different amounts.

- One gram of fat contains 9 calories.
- One gram of carbohydrates contains 4 calories.
- One gram of protein contains 4 calories.

How Your Body Uses Calories

Fat

Let's take a look at this former bad boy and neo-hero. Fat is a necessary part of a well-balanced diet. Fat is essential to live. It protects the internal organs, maintains body temperature, and is a part of all your cells. For women, a good rule of thumb for a minimum amount of body fat would be about 12 percent. Elite athletes often have less. This is a minimum, not the norm. A normal range would be 18 to 26 percent. Pay attention to the way you feel—your energy and moods—not just the way you look or how much you weigh.

How Your Body Uses Fat. If you eat 100 calories of fat, 97 of those calories are stored as fat. Three calories are lost as heat in the transfer. Research shows that the body is more efficient at storing fat calories than at storing carbohydrates. You need this fat as a source of essential fat-soluble vitamins and fatty acids. Fat also helps you feel full and satisfied. Fat is present in most foods, except sugars such as honey and molasses. As a general guideline, you should limit your fat consumption to no more than 30 percent of your daily caloric intake and no less than 20 percent. You should try to eat as many of the good fats as possible.

Fats: Bad and Good. There are three types of fat: saturated, polyunsaturated, and monounsaturated. The difference has to do with the amount of hydrogen ions per molecule. If a fat has all the hydrogen it can hold, it is saturated. If only one hydrogen ion is missing, it is monounsaturated. If several hydrogen ions are missing, it is polyunsaturated.

The Bad Fats. You want to avoid *saturated* fats. They are the villains that raise the dangerous cholesterol—LDL cholesterol. Saturated fats are found primarily in animal products: cheese, whole milk, lard, cream, butter, and fatty meats. Stearic acid, the primary fatty acid found in lean beef and chocolate, does not seem to affect LDL cholesterol. Also, be warned that coconut, cottonseed, and palm oils are saturated fats.

Now for the other villains, *trans fats*. Trans fats are to be avoided as much as possible. Trans fats are common in fried foods, baked goods, margarine, and other processed foods. Trans fats raise your LDL cholesterol (the bad kind) and your triglycerides while reducing your HDL cholesterol (the good kind). The Food and Drug Administration plans to make listing trans fats on food labels mandatory. But this won't go into effect until 2006.

Now that I've scared you, you probably want to know what trans fats are. A trans fat is a liquid oil that has been modified and changed into a solid. This benefits the manufacturer but not your health. You can avoid trans fats by avoiding products that contain hydrogenated or partially hydrogenated oils.

The Good Fats. *Polyunsaturated* fats are found in most plant oils (except palm, coconut, and cottonseed). Some examples are corn oil, peanut oil, safflower oil, soybean oil, and sunflower oil. The other good fat, *monosaturated*, is found in olive oil and canola oil.

To Sum Up. When you replace bad fat (saturated) with good fat (monounsaturated and polysaturated), your LDL cholesterol (the dangerous kind) decreases.

Carbohydrates

Carbs are now the bad boys of the diet world. They used to be the heroes. Do carbs have a tragic flaw? It might be that we love them too much and eat too many of them, especially in the form of sugar. There is nothing inherently wrong with carbohydrates. In fact, carbs are essential to our health. They are also our body's first choice for energy, which was number one on our list of reasons to eat them.

Fat, the former bad boy, is now touted as the new hero in many diets. It seems as if we always have to demonize something. It's a way to sell books, to gain status. But it's never that simple. Fats were never all bad, either. They are also a combination of good and bad.

How Your Body Uses Carbohydrates. Your body doesn't store carbs as easily as it does fat. If you eat 100 calories of carbohydrates, 23 are lost to heat, and the rest are stored in your liver and muscles as glycogen, to meet your energy needs. Only when glycogen stores are full will carbs be stored as fat. We need to eat carbs daily—they are essential for keeping the muscles primed and the brain functioning with efficiency. The bare minimum is approximately 50 grams, or 200 calories, of carbohydrates a day. This minimum is not ideal. If you don't take in enough carbs, your body has to resort to secondary choices as primary energy suppliers. It has to shift to a less efficient Plan B. Many studies recommend that 50 to 60 percent of your diet should come from carbohydrates.

Simple Carbohydrates. There are two types of carbs: simple and complex. Simple carbs are found primarily in sugar, milk, fruit, and some vegetables (potatoes and carrots). They are simple in their chemical structure—just two molecules hook them together. These simple carbs are quickly digested into the bloodstream, causing blood sugar to rise, giving a boost in energy. The problem is that this is often followed by a low. If your carbs are coming from sugar,

you don't receive any nutritional value. If you eat a carrot, you get an energy boost, plus vitamins, antioxidants, and fiber.

Complex Carbohydrates. Complex carbs are made of long strings of molecules instead of just two. You will find complex carbs in whole wheat bread, beans, brown rice, apples, and oatmeal (to name a few).

To Sum Up. Carbohydrates are your body's first and most efficient source of energy and can also be a good source of fiber, vitamins, and antioxidants. Try to eat primarily complex carbs.

Protein

Nobody has ever said anything bad about protein. It hasn't gone through the highs and lows in popularity like carbs and fats—yet overdoing protein could be worse than either of those. Consuming excess protein puts stress on the liver. When the liver has to process this excess, it is taken away from other vital detoxing duties.

How Your Body Uses Protein. Protein is the body's last choice for energy. At rest, the body uses 2 to 5 percent of calories from protein as an energy source. During endurance activities, the body gets 5 to 10 percent of its energy from protein. Protein can be converted into glucose. If you don't consume enough carbs or fats, your body will use protein as an energy source. But this takes it away from other important duties, such as building and repairing muscle and helping in the formation of enzymes and hormones.

As a general guideline, you need between 7 and 9 grams of protein for every 10 pounds of body weight, depending on how hard you're working out. If you weigh 120 pounds, on the upper end you need 108 grams, and on the lower end you need 84 grams.

Don't limit yourself to thinking protein means meat. You can get your protein from a variety of sources. Other good sources of protein are eggs, soy products, beans, and nuts. Ultimately, proteins are designed to rebuild and repair.

In Conclusion

Fats, carbohydrates, and proteins, are how the body receives its essential nutrients and its energy, and how it rebuilds itself, which are the reasons why we eat—besides the pleasure, of course. How we eat should match these needs in proportion. This overview gives you the basics on how the body is designed to use food. It is your fuel. How well you function, physically and mentally, depends on what you put in your body. This is the other key component, along with exercise, that determines—to a great extent—the quality of your life.

DEVELOPING AN EATING PHILOSOPHY

Since eating is so important, you need to develop a personal philosophy. You can't just leave it to chance and mindlessly eat what is put in front of you. This means you have to think and take action. To get you started, I'm going to share with you my personal eating philosophy.

My list of eating commandments is composed of try-tos—not shall-nots. It's hard in our culture with a busy lifestyle to always eat right. It takes as much effort and planning to eat well as it does to get on a work-out program. You need to know the basics and make a commitment to action. Again, the goal is consistency of effort over time. You don't want to eat good food one week, then eat garbage the next.

Eating Skills

Eating with Moderation

Even if you're eating a healthy diet, overeating can sabotage your work. You need to listen to your body and not overeat. This means knowing when to stop eating. Sounds simple, but it's not. The reasons for overeating are often subtle and complicated: We eat for emotional reasons, because a relationship just ended; we eat for psychological reasons, because we're depressed or anxious. We also squelch our appetites because of cultural pressures to be thin.

The challenge is to listen to your body's hunger cues. The following tips will help you connect to these cues:

1. Slow down and really chew and enjoy your food. Don't rush past your body's chance to say, "I'm full."
2. Halfway through your meal, stop and ask yourself, "Am I satisfied?"
3. Eat up to the point of being physically satisfied and stop, even if there's more on your plate. You can snack later.
4. Don't eat until you are stuffed or full. That's too much.
5. Eat when you're hungry. Don't repress your hunger, either.

A Free Food

A good way to stay consistent is to allow yourself one "free food" a day. This means you don't have to completely exclude anything; just have your favorite treats in moderation, and only one a day. Otherwise, the tendency is to become obsessed with the things that are off-limits and to eventually binge on them. This is physically unhealthy, and psychologically it usually creates guilt. Freud believed that you become obsessed with what you repress. He called it "the return of the repressed." With the free-food rule in place, there will be no repression or obsession. Again, this doesn't mean you can eat a whole gallon of ice cream. Have your free food in smaller portions: Split a dessert; have a cookie; have a couple of scoops of frozen yogurt; have a piece of chocolate or a slice of pizza. Nowadays there are also a lot of healthy versions of your favorite snacks.

Drink Water
We looked at why we eat. The other question would be, why do we drink? About 60 to 70 percent of your body is water. Every metabolic reaction in your body involves water. This includes burning fat and other fuels for energy. This is why water is so important. This is why we can live only three days without it. Losing as little as 1 to 2 percent of your body weight in water will cause fatigue; this is why you need to continually replace your fluids.

Since water is so important, why not give it to your body in its pure form instead of drinking soda or other beverages? Your body needs between eight and twelve cups of water a day to take care of its essential needs. So make the effort to keep hydrated with pure water.

A Simple Manifesto: Four Try-Tos
1. Try to cut way down on sugar. Sugar just takes your body through highs and lows. Sugar has no nutrient value—all the calories are empty. When you eat sugar, you are eating calories without a purpose. Sugar won't satisfy your hunger needs. Since sugar has no nutrients, your body keeps sending the hunger cue to be fed. The body wants nutrients. Sugar doesn't answer this call, so the body keeps asking.
2. Try to eat whole foods instead of processed foods. Whole foods have not been depleted and fragmented like processed foods. Whole foods contain all of their nutrients in their natural state. Try to eat these foods fresh (ideally grown locally), as opposed to canned or frozen.
3. Try to eat organic. Organic foods are allowed to go through their natural growing process, giving them a higher nutrient quality. They are also not sprayed with herbicides and pesticides, which contain poisons. Eating whole foods that are grown organically is not new-age. It is actually old-school. It is the way our grandparents farmed and ate.
4. Try to eat a variety of foods from all the food groups, and try to make most of your carbohydrates complex and your fats the good kind.

To Sum Up
Part of the idea of presenting my eating philosophy has been to inspire you to create your own philosophy, to take the time to think about it. You may side with Sears, Atkins, or Ornish. You may create a vegetarian philosophy or lean toward a raw-food

diet. You may follow the USDA food pyramid. You may count calories and figure out your BMG index. Or you might have a consultation with a diet professional. Having an eating philosophy means you have become aware of the choices you're making and why. It's never too late or too early to become a philosopher.

CHAPTER SEVEN

Reader Two:
The Mind

Assignment #4: Goal Setting

PREVIEW: *This section will give you techniques for setting and achieving goals.*

"TO BE OR NOT TO BE"

You've probably heard it since grade school: You've got to have goals. It's one of those phrases that always get tossed out. The purpose of this talk is to get a little more specific about how to set goals. You need to do more than just identify your wish. "I want a slim and toned belly" is just the first step. Most people stop there.

You need to set specific goals that give you a clear direction and motivation along your path. You have to develop a plan. Hamlet knew there was something fishy in Denmark as he struggled with the question of "to be or not to be." It wasn't until he developed a plan that he grew as a person and ultimately achieved his goal.

WHY GOAL SETTING WORKS

- It focuses your attention in a specific way.
- It gives you a way to measure progress.
- It mobilizes your effort in a consistent and specific way.
- It keeps you focused on the big picture as well as on the immediate goal.
- It allows you to evaluate and create new strategies.

THE TWO TYPES OF GOALS

There are two basic types of goals: outcome and performance.

Outcome goals are centered on a specific result, such as

- lowering your body fat by 3 percent
- being able to perform twenty perfect crunches
- doing ninety minutes of cardio a week

Outcome goals are usually clear-cut. Performance goals are about the process. You are not measuring yourself against an objective result. Instead, you are making goals based on where you are now in the process.

Regardless of the type of goal, avoid the compare-and-despair syndrome. Avoid thoughts like "Cindy is so disciplined. She does yoga five times a week, does aerobics every other day, and even weight trains."

Maybe you don't have time to do Cindy's regimen. Maybe you don't want to. You want to spend more time working out, but you also want to spend time with your kids and pursuing other hobbies. Your personality may also be different from Cindy's. You may not like classes and gyms. So for you, a doable first step might be starting the System and buying a yoga tape to do twice a week.

HOW TO SET GOALS

1. Make your goals specific. There's no reality in generalities. Your goals need to be stated in measurable terms. "I want to get my abs in better shape" is too general. A plan would be to start on a specific workout program.
2. Make your goals challenging yet doable. You need to strike a balance between goals that are challenging and goals that are unrealistic. In the beginning, it is better to err on the side of the doable, to gain momentum.
3. Write down your goals. It's not a goal if it's not written down. Writing them down is an action, a commitment. I make my clients sign a contract. Once you've written your goals down, you need to read them daily. Otherwise they're no better than an old dusty journal from a summer vacation. Read them when you're excited about working out and when you're dreading working out. Either way, they'll give you an extra boost. Post your goals somewhere you can see them—someplace that is impossible to avoid.
4. Set goals that match your personality. This is a complex issue. Assignment #8 (page 84) will give you some guidelines.
5. Have a support system. Whenever you're trying to achieve a goal, it's good to have help. You may not be able to go to your normal sources. Your friends and lover may actually try to lure you away from your workouts and urge you to have dessert and another drink. Family and friends with similar goals are always good. And when it comes to your wellness goals, tune out the naysayers.

SETTING LONG-TERM, INTERMEDIATE, SHORT-TERM, AND DAILY GOALS

You need long-term, intermediate, short-term, and daily goals. You're not going to have major changes overnight. That's why you need steps all along the way. Think of the martial arts. You don't start out as a black belt. First you're a white belt, then a yellow, green, brown, blue, and black. You need to think of your progression toward your goal in small steps, so it's not overwhelming.

Your *long-term goal* is your dream. You need to be able to imagine it in your mind's eye.

Your *intermediate goal* is the midpoint of the process. If you had a three-month exercise plan to get ready for the beach, the six-week mark would be your intermediate benchmark.

Your *short-term goals*, on this three-month schedule, could range from one month to a week, depending on how detailed you need to be.

Your *daily goals* are your bread and butter. These little steps will take you to your dream. If it's a technique goal, make it as specific as possible: "Today I'm going to concentrate on holding my peak contraction on each repetition for the allotted time." If it's an eating goal, be just as clear: "For lunch today, I'm going to have a salad with low-fat dressing and a whole wheat roll. For my four o'clock snack, I'll have an apple."

EVALUATE AND ADJUST

At any time, you can stop and evaluate your goals. There's a learning curve in goal setting that revolves around getting to know your body. You have to be willing to adjust your goals up or down. It can be a difficult proposition to adjust them down, because you can feel like a failure. Don't let your ego get in the way. If you push yourself too hard, it will lead to injury or burnout. Either one of these outcomes will leave you much farther from your goal than the adjustment.

Circumstances that you can't control can also make an adjustment necessary. Don't try to force your way through the flu or a cold, an exhaustive project at work, or any other type of crisis. Adjust to the situation. The key is not to stop completely. In almost any situation, you can find fifteen minutes a few times a week to keep up your momentum and relieve stress. Remember, the ultimate goal is consistency over the long haul.

Assignment #5: Getting Motivated

PREVIEW: *The exercises and techniques in this section will give you a set of motivational tools to get you going.*

MOTIVATION

Motivation is a very personal process. There are hundreds of motivational tapes and books, a cable TV system filled with infomercial gurus, and a long line of miracle products. The bottom line is, do what works for you. Ultimately, motivation has to come from deep within. The exercises and techniques in this section will give you a set of tools. You need to become a miner for those personal gold nuggets of motivation that will *inspire* you into action.

> Take your motivation where you can get it. Here are some examples:
>
> - Cut out photos from magazines; let sports heroes inspire you.
> - Let old lovers push you to the next level.
> - Let anger inspire you (work it right out of your body).
> - Schedule a vacation on the beach.
> - Get in shape for your high school reunion.
> - Get in shape for your wedding.
> - Or just do it for the love of it.

MOTIVATION: THE PERSONAL AND THE EXTERNAL

In a nutshell, motivation is the direction and intensity of one's effort. Motivation is a personal thing. Creating motivation is essential to achieving your goals. So it is important for us to get as specific as we can.

Motivation can come from two basic sources: the personal (internal) and the external. Personal motivation comes from mining your needs, goals, and personality. External motivation comes from outside situations and rewards that help your goals become reality.

The trick is finding a balance between the personal and the external—and discovering what is most effective for your personality.

For example, Albert Einstein hated taking tests. He said, "The coercion had such a deterring effect that, after I passed the final examination, I found the consideration of any scientific problem distasteful to me for an entire year." Einstein did science for the love of it. He wanted the motivation to come from within himself, not from some imposed force, like getting an A on a test.

Other people need the challenge to come from outside themselves before they can get motivated. "I'll bet you a thousand dollars that you can't lose twenty pounds." The bet gets this woman on a workout program and a healthy diet. She loses the weight. She starts to feel better. And, yes, she actually starts to enjoy working out. So after she's won the bet, she keeps working out. The reason changes from an external reward to a personal motivation.

In the long run, you'll need flexible and varied motivational techniques to keep you going. Later in this section, I'll give you a variety of techniques.

There was a classic study done by social scientist Edward Denci in the 1960s. He gave two groups of college students Parker Brothers puzzle games. The goal was to put the puzzles together in their proper formation. One group received a dollar for each puzzle they completed in the allotted time. The other group worked on the puzzles without any mention of reward. After a prescribed amount of time, they were given a break. On the puzzle table in front of them, Denci left a pile of current magazines. The participants were observed through a one-way mirror during this break. The amount of time the players worked on the puzzles during the break was the way Denci measured personal versus external motivation. The participants in the reward group spent significantly less time working on the puzzles. They read the magazines. The other group continued to work on the puzzles during the break. They got pleasure out of doing the activity for its own sake.

Paris or Bust

During a consultation with a client, I asked what her goals were. She said she wanted to lose twenty-five pounds. She talked at length about how important this was. She got very upset and confessed that every time she looked in the mirror, she became depressed. As she went over her exercise history, she talked about the frustration of starting a program and then quitting. Even when she stuck with a program, she didn't get the results she wanted. Then she confessed that she really hated working out.

My hunch was that even when she worked out, she just went through the motions. Remember our definition of motivation—motivation is the direction and *intensity* of one's effort. Like this woman, you can stick with a program and still not see results if you don't give it a quality effort. It's about quality and quantity—effort over time.

So I said, "I know you really want to lose twenty-five pounds. Now tell me something else you really want to do." Her eyes lit up. "I've always wanted to go to Europe," she said. "See plays in London. Go to the museums in Paris."

So I made a deal with her: I would train her if, and only if, she would book a vacation to Europe. She didn't think she could afford it. I told her we were going to take off the weight gradually, about a pound a week, so she had six months to save up some money. She waffled.

"So what if you go into a little credit-card debt," I said. "You have a decent job. You can pay it off. What is the choice here: to stay overweight and miserable and never live your dreams, or to get slim and toned and go to Europe?" She pulled out her day planner and we picked out a possible date.

The next week, she signed the contract and bought her ticket. She was motivated and excited. She worked hard, lost the weight, and toured Europe.

The Secret

Let me tell you something—at its highest level, motivation is an action. That's the secret. It's not just a thought in your head. It is an action. You buy the workout book. You sign the contract. You go public and tell your friends your goal. You buy the ticket. You make reservations at your favorite restaurant on the day you get through the System. You take action, and action begets action. That's the way the world works.

My client's case is also an example of creating an external motivation (a trip to Europe) to fulfill a personal desire (to look and feel good). Use this model to achieve your goals.

To Sum Up

Take your motivation where you can get it and let it inspire you each workout. If it's a bet for money, take it. If it's getting ready for weekends at the beach, take it. If it's to show an old boyfriend, take it. In a perfect world, all motivation would be personal and deep. We'd do everything for love. It's not always going to happen. But always keep digging for those deep personal reasons. Also keep giving yourself those rewards, like a dinner out at your favorite restaurant when you've achieved all your goals for the week. Personal and external motivations feed off one another.

STRATEGIES FOR MOTIVATION

- Make sure your long-term, intermediate, short-term, and daily goals are clear. Motivation is directly linked to a plan of action. It's hard to get motivated and stay motivated if you don't know how and why you're doing something.

- Keep your schedule flexible so you don't get stuck in a rut.

- Change your workout when you get bored with it.

- Create rewards for each small goal you achieve. Don't think of just one big reward at the end. If you never get a pat on the back, you lose motivation. These rewards can be as simple as going to a movie, buying a CD, or taking a nap.

- Take time off. When you reach a point of diminishing returns, take a break. A little rest and relaxation is a great attitude adjuster.

- Don't put unnecessary pressure on yourself. Don't base your entire self-worth on this project. Keep things in perspective and make it fun.

Assignment #6: Mind Skills: Relaxation and Performance Techniques

PREVIEW: *In this section, you will learn basic mind skills to help you improve performance and manage stress.*

WORKING OUT YOUR MIND

Your mind responds like a muscle, and you need to train it and use it for it to be in peak condition. This section gives you techniques to control your mind. We'll begin with relaxation techniques. Relaxation is the foundation for performance. You need to be able to quiet your mind and bring it to a point of concentration before you can excel in most activities. Next we'll move to skills that are designed to improve performance. Remember, just like any other skill, the more you practice these techniques, the better you will get.

RELAXATION SKILLS

Relaxation is good. Stress is bad. In our culture, this is a mantra. Yet we all seem to be stressed out. Why is this? Because it needs to be more than talk. You need practical stress-relieving skills. We'll begin with three simple techniques:

Controlled Breathing

One way to achieve a relaxed state is by concentrating on your breathing. Settle in a comfortable position, either lying down or sitting, and focus on inhaling and exhaling for approximately one minute. Then inhale on a count of five and exhale on a count of five. Keep repeating this smooth, regular pattern. Make sure you breathe deeply, letting the breath drop down into your belly so your navel expands.

Focus on feeling the air coming into your lungs and imagine the oxygen being transported to every cell of your body. Every time you breathe out, release on the breath any muscular stress or negative thoughts. Each time you breathe in, imagine the breath purifying your body. Continue this process until you feel relaxed and centered.

This steady, counted deep breathing is a great way to calm your nerves. When you're nervous, your breath is shallow and fast. In fact, if you start to take shallow, fast breaths, you'll begin to feel a little nervous. It's a classic example of the mind-body connection. Deep, steady breaths change this pattern and give your body and mind the message to relax.

Progressive Relaxation

This technique is a way to consciously program your body to relax. You can do it either of two ways. As you move through your body, you can tense and relax each muscle or you can just give the muscle the mental command to relax. In the beginning, it is helpful to tense and relax, so you can clearly feel the difference.

To begin, settle in a comfortable position, either lying down or sitting, and take a couple of deep breaths. Give your body the message to relax. Then start to feel where your body is making contact with the floor or the chair. Now move your focus down to your feet and give them the message to relax, telling all the little muscles on the soles and across the top of your feet to let go. Move up to your calves and give them the message to relax. Move up to your thighs and hamstrings, telling them to relax. Go to the muscles of your buttocks and tell them to relax. Then move to your lower back, middle back, and upper back, giving your entire back, one section at a time, the message to relax. Then send the message to your shoulders, arms, hands, chest, and stomach, telling them to relax. Finish with your neck, head, face, and throat. Tell all the little muscles around your eyes, cheeks, and jaws to relax. Tell your forehead and scalp to relax. After you have given your entire body, part by part, the message to relax, allow yourself to sink deeper into relaxation with each breath, giving in to gravity and melting into the floor or chair.

You can choose to end the relaxation session anytime you wish by simply saying, "On a count of three, I will open my eyes and feel relaxed and energized, ready to go on with my day." This technique is also good to do with a partner. Have him or her talk you through each part of your body.

Meditation

The goal of meditation is simple yet complex. It is about keeping your mind focused and present in the moment, on one task. When your mind resists, you gently bring it back to the moment. Over time, this allows you to be in control of your mind, instead of your mind being in control of you.

A Breathing Meditation

The rules of this meditation are simple. Sit with your back in a straight chair and focus on your breathing—the inhalation and the exhalation. Feel the breath come in through your nose and drop down to your belly, and then feel it completely leave your body through your nose. Also become aware of the natural pause between each inhalation and exhalation. Keep your mind tuned and focused on your breathing process; when your mind wanders, bring it back. This is different from controlled breathing in that you don't have a goal. You allow each breath to be what it is.

THE PERFORMANCE EDGE

The following skills—self-talk, visualization, and focus—are designed to psych you up and help you improve performance:

Self-Talk

We all know the power of positive thinking. You are what you think. Self-talk is what you are saying to yourself or thinking in the moment. The first step is to slow down for a moment and become aware of the tape that is playing in your mind. The second step is to push the stop button and make a new recording.

Being aware of self-talk and becoming proactive in the process will help you to become the ruler of your world. It gives you a choice in how you are going to respond to life's events. We can't control everything, but we can control how we respond to events: We can either move forward or stay stuck in the past.

Self-talk comes in two basic forms: positive and negative. Positive self-talk keeps you focused in the moment and moving forward: "Feel the muscle work. One more rep." Or in a sport, it might be a simple cue like "Keep your eye on the ball" or "Breathe."

Negative self-talk prevents you from taking a new action. It keeps you dwelling on the past moment: "I'll never get my abs in shape." Or in a sport, you might dwell on a bad shot: "That was a stupid shot." Or you might pout, "I'll never be any good," instead of giving yourself positive cues like "Keep your head up. Follow through." Habitual negative self-talk will hold you back in life.

Apply Self-Talk to Exercise

Use self-talk.

1. For motivation on days when you're struggling to work out: "I'll feel so much better after I work out."
2. As a reminder. This is what the Trainer's Tips do. They give you cues to teach and to remind you of the proper technique for the movement with simple phrases like "Hold the peak contraction" and "Control the movement."
3. To maintain good habits. If you have particular bad habits that you struggle with, use self-talk to help break them: "Focus." "Breathe."
4. To push through a workout when you're struggling: "Just one more exercise. Finish strong."

Self-Talk Strategies:
Turn Negatives into Positives

Just because you know about practicing positive self-talk, the negative self-talk isn't going to just magically stop. You need to become a skilled self-talker, turning negative self-talk into positive self-talk. Here are some examples:

Negative: Crunches hurt my neck.
Positive: Just let my arms hold the weight of my head. This will give my neck a break.
Negative: I can't focus today. I have ADD.
Positive: Just breathe and focus on my lower abs.

Self-Talk Basics

1. Keep your statements positive. Positive phrasing: "I will succeed." Negative phrasing: "I will not fail."
2. Keep phrases in the present moment. Present: "I am strong." Not: "I will be strong."
3. Keep it simple. Simple: "No one can stop me." Wordy: "There is no one who can prevent me from reaching my goals."

Visualization

Visualization is the creation of mental pictures. At an unconscious level, you are often creating images. These pictures affect your behavior and influence your actions. The goal of conscious visualization is to create positive images to help you achieve positive goals.

To achieve the abs you want, you have to be able to see them in your mind's eye. You could see them in a still shot, like a picture from a magazine, or you could see them in motion, like a movie in your mind. The most important thing is to see the image in vivid detail. Try to also hook the image up with a feeling. Let the image start to live in your body; let it affect you emotionally; let it inspire you.

Elements of Effective Visualization

1. Ideally, find a quiet place where you won't be disturbed.
2. Start the visualization with controlled breathing or a relaxation technique, to center your body and mind.
3. Use all of your senses to fuel your imagination.
4. Create a scene: Who, what, where, and when.
5. See in specific details, not in generalities.
6. Let the scene affect you emotionally. Feel the emotions run through your body.
7. See how you affect others in your visualization, and how they react to the new you.
8. Practice the visualization process consistently.

Getting Focused and Staying Focused

Focus means paying attention to what is important in your current task and disregarding what is unimportant.

If you're doing crunches, you want to feel your muscles contract and maintain proper technique. You also want to tune out irrelevant thoughts like "What should I have for dinner? I think I'll rent a movie."

You also need to keep your eye from wandering, letting your attention shift to someone walking by or checking out the person exercising next to you.

This is the drama of concentrating, trying to keep your focus on what's important and not letting it drift out of the moment to what is irrelevant.

Four Types of Focus

This breakdown of focus techniques was first pioneered by the sports psychologist R. M. Nideffer. These concentration modes are natural and intuitive, although we are normally not aware of them. Nideffer systemized them, so you can practice them. Your focus, just like looking through the lens of a camera, is what you decide to put your attention on. You can zoom in tight or zoom out to a broader angle. You can look outward or inward, using a broad or narrow focus.

Broad Focus. I also call this soft focus. This is when you take in the whole scene instead of focusing on a specific spot. This is important when you need to see rapid changes in the environment. In sports, a classic example is a fast break in basketball. All the players are running down the court and the woman with the ball has to see the whole court to find the open person or to take it to the hoop herself.

Or let's say you're watching a musical and it's a big dance number. You use a broad focus to see the whole ensemble and the patterns and interactions they create as a group. Then the principle dancer breaks into a solo and you focus just on her.

Narrow Focus. Now as you focus on the principle dancer, your focus zooms in. You are no longer focusing on the whole scene.

External Focus. This is when you focus on something outside yourself. In both of the above examples, the focus was external.

Internal Focus. This is when you focus inward, on your thoughts and feelings.

How the Types of Focus Apply to Exercise

Let's take a set of crunches for an example:

1. You scan the room to place your mat. If you're at home, you check over the room to make sure the space is clear. If you're at the gym, you find a space where you're not in anybody else's way. You are now using a *broad external focus.*
2. You get yourself psyched up with a little pep talk: "All right, let's get one more rep than last time." You are now using a *broad internal focus.*
3. You get ready to begin. You place your fist between your chin and chest for the proper distance between the two. You bring your knees up and check to see if they are directly over your hips. If there is a mirror, you can check to see if your shoulder blades rise off the mat. You are now using a *narrow external focus.*
4. You activate your inner core. As you do your repetitions, you focus on feeling the contraction in the working muscle as you initiate the movement. You are now using a *narrow internal focus.*

To Sum Up

Nideffer's breakdown of focus techniques gives you a systematic way to use concentration when you're working out and in real-life situations. Becoming conscious of how you focus will strengthen each of the concentration modes and make the transition between modes more efficient.

DEVELOP A TRAINING RITUAL

The following is a sample preparation ritual you can use. You may modify it to fit your style.

1. Take a deep breath and get centered, bringing your concentration to the moment and the task at hand.
2. Visualize the exercise you are going to do in perfect form. See the key elements:

   • starting position
   • holding the peak contraction
   • the finish

3. Know the abdominal area you are working, so you can feel the movement initiate from that area.
4. Activate your inner core and begin the exercise.
5. Close out your workout by acknowledging your accomplishments. Every workout is a victory, a step toward your goal. Take a moment to acknowledge your work ethic; then let go and move on with your day.

This preparation will bring you fully to the task. It may sound hokey, but take pride in your technique, as if it were an art form, as if it were ballet.

CHAPTER EIGHT

Reader Three: Know Yourself

Assignment #7: Getting in Touch with Your Exercise Essence

PREVIEW: *This section is about searching for that deep source of motivation I've been talking about.*

CONNECTING TO YOUR EXERCISE ESSENCE

Your *exercise essence* is like your exercise soul. The way to connect to this essence is to use your body in a challenging and invigorating way. To develop your exercise essence,

you need to create a strong connection with your body. Since this partnership is "till death do you part," you might as well make the best of it. This doesn't require years of therapy. It does mean, however, that you need to start a dialogue with your body.

The development of a healthy relationship with your body is the key to sticking with a fitness program and achieving your goals. If there is a secret to looking and feeling good, this is it. It's not the new fitness gadget. It's not a health club membership (the vast majority join, then don't go regularly). It's not some elixir. The secret is building and nurturing a relationship with your body.

Having a weak or superficial connection to your body is one of the primary reasons for quitting an exercise program. It's that simple. If you are going to stay with something over the long haul, you need a deep motivation. This means you need more than a superficial reason for working out. "I want to look good" is okay for starters. We all want to look good. But you need to go deeper.

Starting a Dialogue with Your Body

So let's get to the essence of why you want to work out, giving you a reason to push forward on days you don't feel like it. A deep motivation is a strong current that surges below your daily surface moods and feelings. The first step in this process is a little psychological exercise. The connection that you're going to explore is the hallmark of great athletes in every sport.

Connecting to your essence is about creating a positive and deeply motivated workout habit. To do this, you may have to replace some old habits and ways of thinking with new ones. For athletes, talking with their bodies is an ongoing conversation. If you develop this connection, it will give you payoffs for the rest of your life.

Digging Deep: An Exercise in Discovery

Okay, here's the exercise: You need a notebook, a pen, and a watch. You need to find a quiet place to go and sit. On a sheet of paper, write the categories listed below, leaving several lines of space between each one. Review the examples in the sidebar before you start the exercise.

For each time period, write at least two images or short phrases that describe and evoke a memory about your body and your physical life during that time. You don't have to work in a strict chronological order; go with your instincts. Allow yourself ten minutes to create your list. If you want more time, take it. But stay with it for at least ten minutes. When you're done, keep your list and add to it. Once the pump is primed, memories might start to flow. The following chronology is just a template. Explore memories up to your age.

- Childhood
- Adolescence
- College Years
- Middle Twenties
- Thirties
- Forties
- Fifties
- Sixties
- Seventies and beyond

DIGGING DEEP: IMAGES AND MEMORIES

The following are some examples of images and memories from different people I've had do this exercise.

CHILDHOOD
- relay races at recess
- ballet class
- playing Bombardment in gym class—the only girl who'd play up front with the boys
- obsessive longing for after-school snacks like Oreo cookies, Chips Ahoy!, Devil Dogs, etc.
- lagging at the back of the group during physical-fitness running tests

ADOLESCENCE
- making the field hockey team
- losing interest in ballet
- suddenly having big breasts for my size
- finally menstruating
- only lost weight (and desire for eating) when stressed over relationship with boyfriend

COLLEGE YEARS
- no more organized sports, just a movement or aerobics class here and there
- a year of rehab after a knee injury changed everything—my connection to working out, to my body, increases
- friends and roommates exercised regularly, which motivated me to start running and do exercise classes and tapes
- noticed muscle development in my legs due to regular exercise

MIDDLE TWENTIES
- back to school after injury, depressed, working out went out the window
- eventually got a treadmill, an ab trainer, but use was inconsistent
- first year living on my own, lonely and gained fifteen to twenty pounds
- lost weight when stressed out over a relationship
- stayed thin while in long-term relationship but struggled to maintain physical activity
- decided to finally become a vegetarian

THIRTIES
- gained weight after leaving long-term relationship and living alone again
- noticed subtle body changes, little "saddlebags" developing
- a little butt cellulite started
- wished breasts were perkier
- struggled to reconnect with a physical

life, dabbled in gym memberships, yoga, etc.
- exercised with a trainer, started using weights, and began running and walking regularly; felt myself getting strong
- discovered Pilates

FORTIES
- felt more vulnerable to illness
- concern and confusion about calcium/osteoporosis
- worried about the future effects of menopause on my youthfulness
- looking at a woman in her early twenties, realized I was forty-eight

FIFTIES
- started to lose flexibility
- felt my mortality as I got a mole removed from my arm and checked for cancer
- lost all interest in my body after I got divorced
- slowed down, gained weight
- thoughts about liposuction almost every day

SIXTIES
- Overweight and miserable, I realized I could turn into my mother and live to be ninety; that's thirty years of misery. I started walking and doing an exercise tape.
- I realized at sixty-five that age isn't the sole determinant of being young or old, as I looked at my medal for the triathlon I finished.

Seeing Trends

The second part of the exercise is to look for major trends in your images and memories. Write out each trend in a sentence or two. You may have only one major trend. Some of you may have two or three or more. There's no right or wrong here.

Then describe what your relationship with your body is like right now.

TRENDS: FROM THE PAST TO THE PRESENT

The following examples are of two opposite scenarios. Your relationship with your body might resemble one of these trends or it might be a combination of the two.

EXAMPLE ONE

Past Trends: My activity level has probably always been a good barometer for my mental state/mood. I'm more prone to be lethargic and unmotivated if I'm depressed or going through a crisis.

The Present: I'm feeling kind of "reactivated" by finding a system I like in Pilates that's invigorating but not exhausting. I feel fortunate that I haven't been too prone to body-image problems and that my body seems to have held up despite long inactive periods.

Body Lesson: I need to change the dynamic between my mental state and working out, and let being physical help me feel better instead of letting upsets shut me down. I realize that when I was younger, sports and exercise were a fun and important part of my life. For various reasons, once a structure for that was gone, I let it slip away. Remembering how beneficial it was for me, I'd like to reconnect with it now and make it a part of my life again.

EXAMPLE TWO

Past Trends: My obsessive eating has always been linked to periods in which I've struggled with loneliness, feelings of inadequacy, and self-dissatisfaction. I have often tried to incorporate exercise into my life but have rarely been able to make it stick for more than a few months at a time.

The Present: Becoming more aware of my patterns regarding eating and exercising and my emotions has helped me start to keep bad habits in check. Having someone to partner with has always motivated me and helped me to maintain an exercise schedule, so I have sought out a friend to take classes with.

Body Lesson: Perhaps turning to exercise during difficult times—rather than to food—could be helpful in curbing obsessive thinking about food and would reduce the stress that triggers it.

Q and A with Your Body

The final step in connecting to your exercise essence is to start a dialogue with your body, a little question-and-answer session. Begin with these questions, then let your body respond. The key questions are numbered. They will help give your dialogue structure. Let the conversation go where it wants to go, but keep these key questions in mind.

Sample Dialogue

1. *You:* How are you feeling?
   Body: Pretty good.
2. *You:* What would make you feel better?
   Body: Stretch more. And let's get outside more, hike and run. The treadmill is okay, but how about a nice wooded trail?
   You: Okay.
   Body: I'm not done. I always feel tight, especially in my back. And I need more water. I would just feel cleaner if I had a lot of fresh water. And one more thing: Eat more vegetables. I like pasta, but at every meal?

3. *You:* Do I do anything that upsets you?
   Body: Yeah.
   You: What?
   Body: You don't really pay attention to me when you're supposed to be paying attention to me.
   You: Like when?
   Body: Like when we're working out. You're thinking about other things instead of concentrating on what we're doing. It's like you're not really present.
4. *You:* I'll work on that. Where do you want us to be ten years from now?
   Body: Flexible and strong. I want to be limber and have good posture. Not be some hunched, middle-aged woman who can't take care of herself.
5. *You:* Okay. How about in one year?
   Body: I'd like to be cooking more and be in a regular class like yoga or a martial art. Try something new. But still keep with our basic workout.
6. *You:* How about a month from now?
   Body: I want to really analyze my weaknesses and start to work on them. Because problem areas are just going to accelerate as I get older.
   You: What do you want to do about it?
   Body: Find a yoga studio and go twice a week.
   You: It's a deal.

Try to wrap up this first conversation with a friendly negotiation. Make a contract, a firm promise outlining how you're going to work together to achieve your goals. Write out this contract and the terms of your agreement.

Contracts can be renegotiated and challenged, but don't break off the agreement without a dialogue. Never ignore what your body has to say or shut your body out of the negotiation process. This will be the beginning of a beautiful relationship.

Your body may ask a lot of you. Tell her you can't do it all at once. You can't change your lifestyle overnight. See the sidebar for a sample contract that came out of the dialogue just presented.

THE CONTRACT

I agree over the next month to do the following two things.

1. Drink more water.
2. Sign up for a yoga class and attend at least once a week, maybe twice.

After six weeks, we can address some of the other issues.

[Your signature]

Going Deeper

Starting a dialogue with your body may be filled with small talk at the start. After all, you're just getting to know each other. In the beginning, you may apologize for stuffing down too many slices of pizza, but if you stay with it, the dialogue will get deeper. As trust develops, more essential questions about the way you live may enter the dialogue. Your body may tell you changes have to be made or there will be breakdowns. The messages it sends you will be simple and clear:

- Drink less coffee and alcohol.
- Get more sleep.
- Take a yoga class if you want to be able to tie your shoes pain-free and keep your golf score down.
- Life is not all about money and work.

Or your body may inspire you with a challenge: "I'm not over the hill. I want to be active: hike, ski, and play tennis. So let's get it together, so we can do the things we love long after retirement."

In the course of these dialogues, your body will share its wisdom with you. It's up to you to listen and translate this wisdom into action.

Assignment #8: Knowing Your Personality Type

PREVIEW: *This section will help you discover your personality type and discusses how it relates to exercise.*

KNOW YOURSELF: PERSONALITY-TYPE INTRODUCTION

Part of being a personal trainer is being a psychologist. But when it comes to designing a workout program, this seldom gets talked about. It's my job as a trainer to quickly discover what will work and what won't. This section will give you some tips and guidelines for discovering and working with your own personality traits.

Before we get into the personality types, let's go over some basics. First of all, each type is just a simple outline of dominant characteristics. Everyone is a combination of different types. Each of us has a social and reclusive side. The pairs give you a way of thinking about yourself and your tendencies. This section is only a short introduction—your personality is complex, not one-dimensional. The goal of this section is to give you a way to start to connect your personality with working out.

It is also important to understand that a value judgment is not being placed on one type above another. Each type has its own style of trying to achieve a similar end.

BASIC TYPES

Solo or Social
These two types explore how you relate to the world. When thinking about these two, ask yourself what you do to recharge and relax. This doesn't mean you have to be either a party animal or a loner.

Solo. She likes to be alone or with a close friend to recharge.

Social. She likes to go to parties or be in other social situations to relax and recharge.

Workout Strategy. If you know your type, it's easy to choose a workout plan. If you're the social type, take classes. If you're the solo type, you should train alone or with a close friend. Get a tape instead of taking a class. This is common sense, but you would be surprised how many people choose a workout plan that goes against their personality. The result is predictable. The person loses motivation to stick with the program.

It's also fine to mix it up. Sometimes you want to be alone; other times you want to be around people. Listen to your needs.

Step-by-Step or the Big Picture
These two types explore your learning style.

Step-by-Step. She likes to learn things one step at a time and to understand the reasons that connect each step. She likes concrete facts, details, and specific instructions.

The Big Picture. She likes to see the whole first, to understand the larger concepts, the general patterns, before filling in the details.

Workout Strategy. A lot of the information I'm giving you in this book is practical, detailed, and step-by-step. This organized structure is an inherent part of a how-to book. For example, this book suggests keeping a workout log and journal. But this type of detail work and specificity might drive the Big Picture type insane. It may grind against her nature, making her quit the program. So the workout log is not for her. Know this and don't let it drive you off the program. Don't turn it into some kind of strike against your character, thinking you're a failure. It's just not for you. Recognize this and move forward.

This book is also designed for the Big Picture type. That's why the program is at the front of the book instead of at the end, after a bunch of information. So jump right in and fill in the important details as you go.

For the Step-by-Stepper, the log and journal can be a source of motivation and structure. The program is also designed in a step-by-step fashion so you don't get frustrated.

Know your learning style and let it work for you, not against you.

The Planner or Go with the Flow

These two types explore how you structure your life and make your decisions.

The Planner. She likes things clearly ordered and mapped out for the day.

Go with the Flow. She likes to take things as they come instead of having a firm plan.

Workout Strategy. Okay, we know what the Planner needs. We know the virtues of being well organized and having a clear vi-

sion. This is a skill we all need to move ahead in the world, and we all have it in different degrees. This book follows that philosophy. To have a plan is not that much different from having a dream. We all have dreams. To the Planner, I say keep it up, but also be careful. Don't let your planning turn into a rigid compulsion. You have to be open to taking a detour. You have to listen to your body; it may need a break. Being too rigid can lead to burnout and injury.

Now to Go with the Flow. If your type needs to go with the flow, a strict routine is a surefire recipe for getting discouraged and quitting the program. Variety and change are important training principles. But as I did with the Planner, I will give you a word of warning. You need to keep some consistency and structure to get results, especially in the beginning. You need to learn the basic techniques and build a foundation. The single most important reason for this is safety. Proper technique and a base of strength are key for preventing injury. This means you must stay with the plan, learn the basics, and build a foundation on a schedule. So, the early stages, getting through the System, may be your biggest challenge.

Now for the good news. Once you get through the System and have a foundation, you can start to vary your workout as your heart tells you. The more advanced you get, the more you can follow your instincts and go with the flow.

These types are related to the head and heart. The head wants to be rational and plan things out. The heart wants to go with how it feels. They need to temper each other. The head needs some kind of plan, a clear dream to get what it wants. And every plan, to be successful, needs a big heart behind it.

TO SUM UP

Working out is a way to get to know not only your body but also your mind. The key is knowing your tendencies, so you can channel them to work for you.

Assignment #9: Knowing Your Body Type

PREVIEW: *This section will help you discover your body type and discusses how it relates to exercise.*

KNOW YOURSELF: BODY-TYPE INTRODUCTION

You need to know yourself inside and out: You need to know your exercise essence and your personality type, and you need to know your body's structure, its type.

First, I want to say that looking at body types can create anxiety. It always does with me. As I look at the three types—ectomorph, mesomorph, and endomorph—my heart starts to race a little. For me, this comes from its harsh objective nature. The voice echoes in my mind, "This is what I am and there's nothing I can do about it." Nobody likes to be typed. It can make you feel limited and constrained and misunderstood.

So, let me say this. These types are just examples for reference and guidance. No one is a pure type. We are all combinations to a greater or lesser degree. When you analyze yourself, you need to look at what is your prominent type in the mixture. Knowing your body will help you set training goals and design a personal program. Knowing your predominant type will help you make commonsense adjustments in your training. Self-knowledge and self-exploration can always be a little unsettling. But as Socrates said, "The unexamined life is not worth living."

TRAINING YOUR TYPE

After a description of each type, I will give basic workout guidelines. I want to stress again that most of us are mutts, a mix of body types. So, the recommendations I'm giving are for the prominent type in your mix. Second, for every body type, I would recommend a complete workout that includes strength, cardio, and flexibility programs. My guidelines are tweaks on this approach, changes you might make within a given program.

Also, these guidelines are for basic programs. The more advanced you become, the more you need to ratchet up your workouts. The guidelines will give you an idea of where you need to place your emphasis. Ultimately, this will depend on your individual goals. A mesomorph, who puts on muscle easily, may want to emphasize lifting to improve performance in a sport or because she's decided to enter a local bodybuilding contest. Another meso may want to de-emphasize putting on muscle, which is already a strong point, and focus more on cardio.

You can shape your body through training. You are not helpless to make changes in your body, regardless of your prominent type.

THE THREE BODY TYPES

Ectomorph

She is naturally low in body fat, thin and lean, with a fast metabolism. Her body is shaped by vertical lines. She has problems gaining weight and putting on muscle. If she wanted to be a runway model and was the right height, she could go to New York and give it a shot. An ectomorph doesn't have to be five feet ten inches; she can be any height.

Celebrity examples: Naomi Campbell, Cameron Diaz, Nicole Kidman, Gabrielle Reece.

Training Guidelines

Strength. Weight training should be an important part of your regimen, since it focuses on a weak area. You can stay in the eight- to twelve-repetition range, but you can work up to three sets per exercise. Since your goal is strength, rest one to two minutes between sets, so your muscles can recuperate.

Cardio. Take classes that combine cardio with strength work. Body-sculpting classes are great for your type.

Stretching. Take yoga classes that also emphasize strengthening moves.

Eating. Since you have a fast metabolism, it's important that you consume enough healthy calories. Small healthy snacks between meals is a good strategy.

Mesomorph

She has an athletic, muscular body, a longish torso with a full chest. The mesomorph's body is shaped by angular lines. She has narrow, powerful hips and broad shoulders. She builds muscles easily and carries a little more body fat than an ectomorph. Being in the middle, her body takes on the tendencies of both ectos and endos. She has a slower metabolism than an ecto, but it is faster than an endo's. She gains muscle faster than an ecto, but not as fast as an endo. Again, like all the types, this body can come in any size, from petite to large.

Celebrity examples: Halle Berry, Mia Hamm, Madonna, Lucy Liu.

Training Guidelines

Strength. Since your type is muscular and gains strength more easily than an ecto, you can do just one set of each exercise. You can stay in the eight- to twelve-repetition range.

Cardio. Since you are prone to carry a higher percentage of fat, cardio is a key

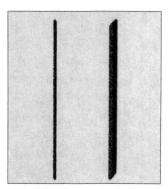

ECTOMORPH

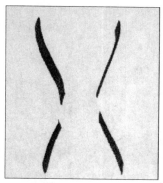

MESOMORPH

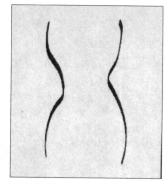

ENDOMORPH

component for you. Try to do four cardio sessions a week. Mix it up: walk, run, bike, use your favorite gym machine.

Stretching. Doing a general hatha yoga class or tape three times a week would be great for you.

Eating. A healthy diet and regular exercise should keep you at an optimal body weight. You will get into trouble if you overeat and underexercise.

Endomorph

She is larger boned and her body is shaped by curved lines. She carries a higher fat percentage, has a slower metabolism, and gains weight easily. She also gains muscle and strength easily.

Celebrity examples: Anna Nicole Smith, Catherine Zeta-Jones, Mary Lou Retton, Drew Barrymore.

Training Guidelines

Strength. Since your type is muscular and gains strength more easily than ectos and mesos, you can do just one set of each exercise. But you should train at a higher repetition scheme. Work your upper-body exercises between twelve and sixteen reps, and your lower-body exercises between fifteen and twenty reps.

Cardio. Since you are prone to carry a higher percentage of fat and have a slower metabolism, cardio should be the center of your program. Try to do five cardio sessions a week. Mix it up: Walk; run; bike; use your favorite gym machine. Aim for forty-minute sessions.

Stretching. Doing a general hatha yoga class or tape three times a week would be a good base. Then try to alternate with a more intense power-yoga routine or a Bikram class.

Eating. If you are predominantly endo, you will have to be more disciplined with food intake and working out in order to keep your body weight down.

TO SUM UP

Knowing your predominant body type will help you train to achieve a balance, focusing on your weak areas and maintaining your strengths.

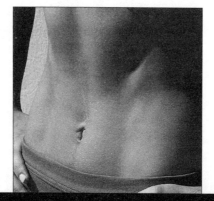

PART FOUR

Wellness

In this part you learn the basics of applying wellness concepts to your life. The emphasis will be on physical wellness. You will be given basic programs for flexibility, strength training, and aerobic fitness.

CHAPTER NINE

Wellness Basics

PREVIEW: *In this chapter you will learn how to analyze your life using the basic concepts of wellness.*

What Is Wellness?

Complete wellness is a lifestyle. It centers on your ability to take responsibility for how you live and the choices you make. Wellness means taking an active role in improving every aspect of your life in order to achieve a productive, healthy lifestyle.

Abdominal development is an important part of physical wellness, but it is only one element, along with strength training, cardio work, and a stretching program. And exercise wellness is just one piece of your complete wellness profile. This chapter will give you an overview of life beyond great abs. It will introduce the six dimensions of wellness.

The Six Dimensions of Wellness

There are six major dimensions of wellness: physical, emotional, spiritual, intellectual, social, and vocational. The choices you make in developing these dimensions will reflect the type of lifestyle you lead. Being aware of these choices is your first step to balance.

Physical development emphasizes choices that create a healthy body. These include daily exercise, diet, and medical care. They also include the use and abuse of tobacco, drugs, and alcohol.

Emotional development emphasizes awareness and acceptance of your feelings. An emotionally well person maintains satisfying relationships with others, while feeling positive and enthusiastic about his or her own life. She also maintains minimal levels of stress, develops healthy feelings, and uses nondestructive emotional outlets.

Spiritual development is the quest for meaning and purpose. A spiritually well person develops, evolves, and practices his or her religious, political, environmental, and personal beliefs.

Intellectual development encourages creative, stimulating mental activities. An intellectually well person uses all resources and knowledge available to improve skills, while expanding potential for sharing with others. Intellectual stimulation and learning are crucial elements in adapting to change.

Social development encourages contributing to the human community and physical environment. A socially well person emphasizes interdependence with others, with nature, and with his or her own family. A socially well person has developed healthy ways to interact with, react to, and live with other people involved in his or her life.

Vocational development encourages growth and happiness in your work. A vocationally well person seeks jobs that give personal satisfaction and enrichment.

THE WEB OF WELLNESS

To understand complete wellness, we should look at these dimensions as if they were part of a pie chart, a pie chart that is divided into six even slices representing the six dimensions of wellness. Each piece of the pie is important to the whole. A complete pie chart with all the pieces fitting together shows a healthy wellness profile. If one piece of pie has a problem, it will affect all the other pieces.

For example, if you recently fell and broke your ankle, your physical wellness would be taxed. If your job requires you to be active and/or you missed work due to your injury, your vocational wellness would also be affected. Emotionally, you would also be stressed because of the injury. And because of your greater dependency on family and friends, your social component would also be affected. Everything intermingles to create that web of wellness.

Everyone's Different

It's important to understand that not everyone's pie chart will look the same. For instance, a professor may have a larger piece of pie for intellectual stimulation than a massage therapist, who works more intuitively and physically. An athlete would have a larger piece of pie for physical issues than a minister of a church, whose religious beliefs are the substance of his or her life. Each one of our pie charts will look different, with emphasis on the things that make us different.

Make Your Own Pie Chart

The divisions of your pie chart will directly reflect how much importance each of the six dimensions has for you. Look at dividing

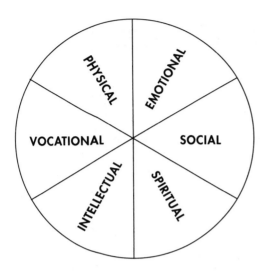

your chart on a percentage basis. Out of the 100 percent, how important are the different dimensions? For example: 30 percent importance on physical wellness, 20 percent importance on vocational wellness, 13 percent importance on social, 13 percent emotional, 13 percent intellectual, and 11

percent on spiritual wellness. It's difficult to place a numerical value on these dimensions, but this kind of introspection will lead to valuable self-knowledge.

The Physical Dimension

Since this is a book about abs, let's look more closely at physical well-being, specifically exercise wellness.

Just as you created your overall wellness profile, you can also create a profile of your *physical wellness.* Within the *physical wellness* piece of pie, we will focus on three elements: stretching, cardio work, and strength training. There are many benefits of exercise: stress reduction, weight loss, cardiovascular benefits, muscular strength, endurance, and increased flexibility. To achieve these benefits, however, you need a complete fitness program. The next chapter will help you get started on a complete program.

CHAPTER TEN

The Complete Program: Stretching, Cardio, Weight Training

PREVIEW: *In this chapter you will learn basic routines for stretching, cardio work, and weight training.*

Getting Started

It is important that you begin your comprehensive exercise program slowly and increase your exercise levels only as you feel comfortable. The goal of the programs in this chapter is to get you started. They are the first step, the building of a foundation, the creating of a habit. How you ease into the Complete Program will depend on your goals and how much time you can commit. The entire program will take one hour and you need to do it three times a week. The breakdown looks like this:

- ten minutes of stretching
- thirty minutes of cardio
- twenty minutes of lifting

Before you start the program, make sure you check with your doctor.

STRATEGIES

There are lots of ways to work this program into your life:

- Start out doing the Complete Program twice a week. You will still look and feel better even if you can only commit to twice a week, as long as you stay with it over the long haul.
- Break it up. You can alternate days. For example:

Monday: Cardio
Tuesday: Weight training and stretching
Wednesday: Cardio
Thursday: Weight training and stretching
Thursday: Cardio
Friday: Weight training and stretching

- For example, maybe you are already doing a yoga class two or three times a week. Then you wouldn't need to do the stretching program. You would want to put your focus on weight training and cardio work.

You can also start out by adding just one element of the program at a time. If you start to do just thirty minutes of cardio a day, that's big. The main thing is, you need to start thinking about the big picture—a complete fitness plan.

Stretching: Basic Moves

Stretching works the muscles, ligaments, and joints. Flexibility is important in maintaining posture, joint mobility, and range of motion, and it helps keep the ligaments and tendons from tightening. Stretching needs to be done at least three times a week and should involve all the major muscle groups and joints. Stretching at the end of a workout is a good way to cool down and safely improve your flexibility when your body is warm.

GUIDELINES

- You should start slow and stay within your comfort zone, breathing into the stretch.
- Stretch only until you feel slight discomfort (not pain!).
- Then hold the position, without bouncing, for the recommended time.

The Stretches

ELONGATION: Lie flat on your back with your arms fully extended over your head and your legs fully extended on the floor. Extend from your fingertips to your toes, lengthening your entire body in both directions. Hold for 10 seconds.

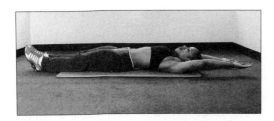

KNEES-TO-CHEST HUG: Lie flat on your back and bring both knees to your chest. From this position, grab your lower legs just below the knee and gently hug your knees to your chest. Keep your neck lengthened. Hold for 20 seconds.

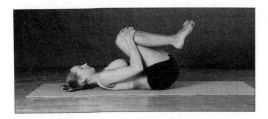

HAMSTRING: Lie flat on your back with your knees bent and both feet on the floor. Grab your right leg below your knee, at your hamstring, then straighten the leg. Gently pull it toward your head. Straighten out your left leg if you can do so without pain. Hold for 20 seconds. Repeat stretch with your left leg.

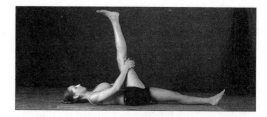

KNEES-TO-SIDE: Lie flat on your back with your knees bent and both feet on the floor. Let both legs fall to one side. Return to the starting position and let your legs fall to the other side. Hold for 15 seconds on each side.

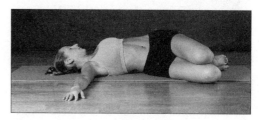

BACK ARCH: Lie on your stomach with your hands, palms down, under your chest. Slowly arch your back, using your arms to gently press your torso up. Your back muscles do most of the work; use your arms just to increase your range of motion. Lift your chin and look up. Slowly lower your torso back to the starting position. Hold for 10 seconds.

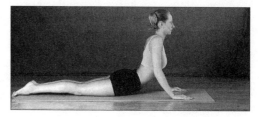

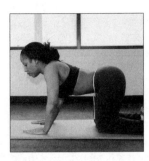

DOWN CAT—UP CAT: Begin on all fours with a flat back—your hands under your shoulders and your knees under your hips. Arch your back up like an angry cat, lowering your head to look out between your legs. Hold for 5 seconds.

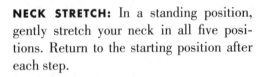

Then arch your back in the opposite direction, looking up and raising your chin. Hold for 5 seconds.

Repeat the sequence 3 times.

NECK STRETCH: In a standing position, gently stretch your neck in all five positions. Return to the starting position after each step.

STARTING POSITION: Align your head with your spine, eyes looking straight ahead.

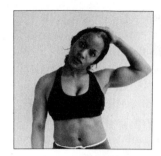

POSITION TWO: Lower your left ear to your left shoulder. Hold for 10 seconds.

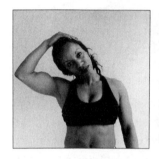

POSITION THREE: Look straight ahead, then lower your right ear to your right shoulder. Hold for 10 seconds.

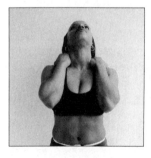

POSITION FOUR: Lengthen your neck as you slowly and gently drop your head backward. Hold for 10 seconds.

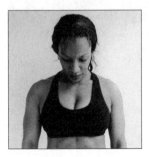

POSITION ONE: Lower your head forward, chin to chest. Hold for 10 seconds.

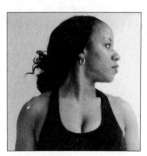

POSITION FIVE: Turn your head to each side, looking as far over each shoulder as possible. Hold for 10 seconds.

SHOULDER ROLL: In a standing position, raise your shoulders toward your ears and then roll them backward. Repeat the move-

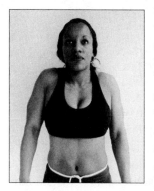

ment, but this time raise your shoulders and roll them forward. Then bring your shoulders up toward your ears and hold for a count of three and release. Repeat 5 times.

Cardiovascular Fitness

Cardiovascular fitness is achieved by performing activities that tax the heart, lungs, and circulatory system. When cardiovascular exercise is performed, it puts a demand on the oxygen-exchange systems of your body. Oxygen is taken from the lungs into the circulatory system, then distributed to the muscles that are being used during exercise. The oxygen is then used to help break down the stored fats into energy for the working muscles. This exchange system forces the lungs and heart to become extremely efficient so that the working muscles can continue their activities.

The American College of Sports Medicine states that thirty minutes of cardiovascular exercise at least three times a week is sufficient to produce significant health benefits. A cardiovascular program consists of activities that allow you to reach 65 to 85 percent of your maximum heart rate for a duration of no less than twenty minutes. Popular cardio exercises are walking, jogging, swimming, bicycling, and aerobic classes (step, Tae Bo).

FINDING YOUR TARGET HEART RATE

The following formula will determine your target heart rate. For an example, let's use someone who is thirty years old.

At birth, your maximum heart rate is 220 beats per minute. Each year you age, your maximum heart rate decreases by 1 beat. So to determine your maximum heart rate, you subtract your age from 220. If you are thirty, your maximum heart rate is 190 beats a minute.

For training purposes, your target zone is between 65 and 85 percent of your maximum heart rate. By target zone, I mean the rate at which you want your heart to be beating to get the desired training effect.

The most practical way to test this during a workout is to figure out your ten-second pulse rate. The way to do this is to multiply your maximum heart rate (220 minus your age) by 0.65 and 0.85, and then divide those figures by 6 (because there are six 10-second periods in every minute). The two resulting figures are the low and high ends for your target zone. When working out, you want to keep your heart rate between these parameters.

$$220 - 30 = 190 \text{ beats per minute}$$
(Maximum heart rate)

$$190 \times 0.65 = 123.5 \text{ beats per minute}$$
(Lower end of target)

$$190 \times 0.85 = 161.5 \text{ beats per minute}$$
(Upper end of target)

In the example above, you want to be between twenty-one and twenty-seven beats in the ten-second count. These are your lower and upper target pulses for ten seconds during exercise. In the middle of your exercise session, count your number of heartbeats in ten seconds by checking your pulse at your wrist or on your neck. It should be somewhere between the upper and lower ends of your target pace.

CARDIOVASCULAR PROGRAM GUIDELINES

The following guidelines are for a progressive cardiovascular program. The program gradually eases you into aerobic training. You want to start slow and build a foundation. If you need to take more time at any level, that's fine; move at your own pace.

Level One: Weeks One and Two

5-minute easy pace
5-minute target pace
5-minute easy pace
Total time: 15 minutes

Level Two: Weeks Three and Four

5-minute easy pace
5-minute target pace
2-minute easy pace
5-minute target pace
5-minute easy pace
Total time: 22 minutes

Level Three: Weeks Five and Six

5-minute easy pace
10-minute target pace
2-minute easy pace
10-minute target pace
5-minute easy pace
Total time: 32 minutes

Level Four: Weeks Seven and Eight

5-minute easy pace
15-minute target pace
2-minute easy pace
15-minute target pace
5-minute easy pace
Total time: 42 minutes

Level Five: Maintenance

5-minute easy pace
10- to 30-minute target pace
5-minute easy pace
Total time: 20 to 40 minutes (depending on how long you stay in the target zone)

Weight Training

Weight, or strength, *training* provides increased strength gains and increased endurance for your muscles, joints, bones, and ligaments. The kinds of benefits achieved with weight training include better posture, stronger structural features, stronger bones, increased strength for daily activities, improved muscle tone, and flexibility and strength in your joints.

A complete weight-training program includes exercises designed for all the major muscle groups. The program should be performed two to three times a week. Weight training can be done a variety of ways: with free weights or strength machines, or through other kinds of resistance training methods.

You should train your larger muscle groups first, followed by your smaller muscles.

BASIC WEIGHT-TRAINING PROGRAM

The following program is a basic routine that works all your major muscle groups. It is a good beginner's routine. The goal is to build a solid foundation so you can go to the next level. The routine was designed using minimal equipment (all you need is a set of dumbbells) so you can do it at home or at the gym. It is important to perform the exercises in the order given.

GUIDELINES

- Complete this routine two or three times a week.
- For upper-body exercises, stay within a ten- to fifteen-repetition scheme. This means choosing a weight that will allow you to do at least ten reps. When you work your way up to fifteen repetitions, add weight. Continue this progressive cycle of adding weight.
- For lower-body exercises (squats and lunges), work up to fifty reps. For lunges, that would mean twenty-five on each side.
- Work up to forty pushups.
- If you want to devote more time to weight training, after four weeks add an extra set to each exercise.
- Apply all the techniques you learned in Chapter Two, "Ab Basics": breathing, controlled movement, focusing the mind.

The Routine: The Basic Eight

Body Area: Chest

■ Pushups

STARTING POSITION: Lie on your stomach with your legs extended, your toes tucked, your elbows bent, and your hands placed outside of and even with your shoulders. Straighten your arms, lifting your entire body off the floor and balancing on your hands and your toes.

THE MOVE: Lower your body, letting your chest make contact with the floor. Then straighten your arms, raising your body back to the starting position. This is one repetition.

VARIATION: This exercise can also be done from your knees. Bend your knees so your lower legs are up in the air and you're balancing on your hands and the muscles just above your knees. Then lower your body.

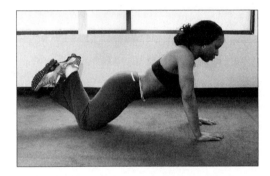

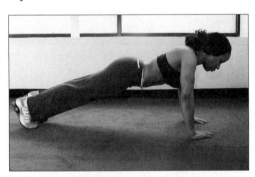

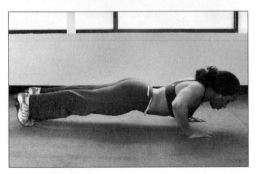

TRAINER'S TIPS

- Think of your body as a solid unit, moving as a whole.
- Keep your head and neck in alignment with your spine, looking straight down, not up.
- Concentrate on your chest muscles as you go through the entire range of motion.
- Extend your arms until they are just short of locking out.
- Exhale as your push up; inhale as you go down.

The Routine: The Basic Eight

Body Area: Back

■ Bent Rows

STARTING POSITION: Holding a dumb-bell with your right hand, step forward with your left leg. Then, bending forward at your waist and using your left arm for support, create between a 45- and 90-degree angle with your upper body. Let your right arm hang down, palm facing in.

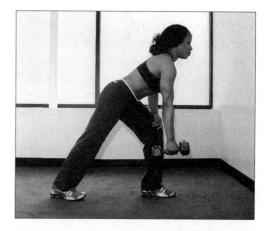

THE MOVE: Using your back muscles, pull the dumbbell to your chest. Then lower it in a controlled motion. Repeat the movement with your left hand and right leg.

TRAINER'S TIPS

- Imagine you have a string on your elbow and the movement is initiated from there, instead of your hand pulling.
- Focus on pulling with your back muscles.
- Control the motion for both phases of the movement; don't let gravity take over.
- Exhale as you pull the weight toward your chest. Inhale as you lower the weight.

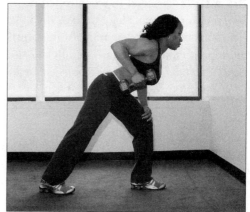

The Routine: The Basic Eight

Body Area: Legs

■ Squats

STARTING POSITION: Prepare to squat by first setting your lower body: feet comfortably apart (shoulder-width in most cases), toes pointed slightly out, knees unlocked, and your weight distributed from the balls of your feet to your heels. Next, set your upper body: chest out, shoulders back, lower back neither curved nor rounded, head in alignment with your spine, eyes looking straight ahead, and your arms extended out in front of your body.

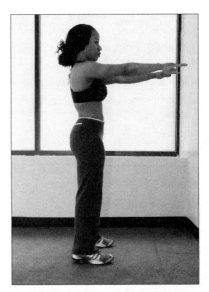

THE MOVE: Descend in a controlled manner (your hips moving backward as if you're sitting and your torso leaning forward), until the tops of your thighs are parallel to the floor. Don't let your knees come out over your toes. Return to the starting position.

TRAINER'S TIPS

- You can add weight by holding dumbbells at your sides.
- Don't bounce at the bottom of the movement.
- Keep your heels flat.
- Don't allow your hips to sway backward as you come up.
- Focus your mind on your thigh muscles.

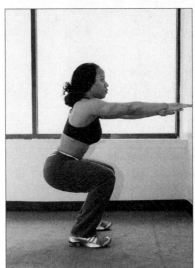

The Routine: The Basic Eight

Body Area: Legs

■ Lunges

STARTING POSITION: Prepare to lunge by first setting your lower body: feet shoulder-width apart, toes pointed straight ahead, knees slightly bent, and weight distributed evenly on your feet. Next, set your upper body: chest out, shoulders back, lower back neither arched nor rounded, head in alignment with your spine, eyes looking straight ahead. Then step forward with your right leg.

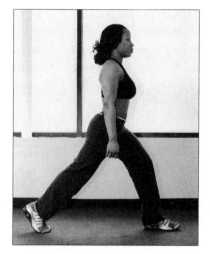

THE MOVE: Lower your body, letting your back knee touch the floor. Do not let the knee of your front leg extend over your toes. Your back leg should be under your hip. Push back with your front leg to return to the starting position. Repeat all the reps with the same leg or alternate legs.

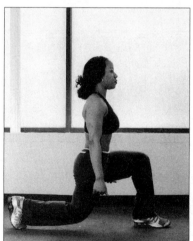

TRAINER'S TIPS

- You can add weight by holding dumbbells at your sides.
- Keep your back and neck aligned.
- Make sure your hips drop straight down rather than sway forward.
- Don't bounce your knee off the floor.
- Your eyes should look straight ahead throughout the movement.

The Routine: The Basic Eight

Body Area: Shoulders

■ Rotation Press

STARTING POSITION: Sit on the edge of a bench or stand with your feet shoulder-width apart and your knees unlocked. Hold both dumbbells underneath your chin with your hands rotated so your palms face your body.

THE MOVE: As you raise both dumbbells directly over your head, rotate both hands so that your palms face away from your body when your arms are fully extended. Bring both dumbbells together at the top as you straighten your arms. Return to the starting position in a controlled motion.

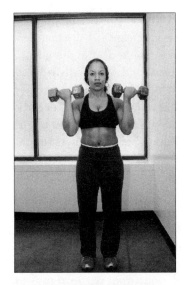

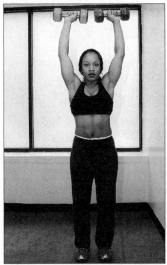

TRAINER'S TIPS

- Maintain good posture throughout the exercise.
- Avoid arching your lower back as you lift.
- Keep your elbows aligned with your ears.
- Focus your mind on your shoulders throughout the exercise.

The Routine: The Basic Eight

Body Area: Upper Back (Trapezius) Muscles

■ Shrugs

STARTING POSITION: Stand with your knees slightly bent, holding two dumbbells at your sides, palms facing in.

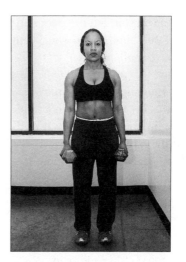

THE MOVE: Keeping proper back alignment (back straight, chest out, eyes straight ahead), elevate the dumbbells by raising your shoulders toward your ears. Return to the starting position in a controlled motion.

TRAINER'S TIPS

- Focus on raising your shoulders, not using your arms and hands.
- Don't come up on your toes.
- Let your arms and shoulder blades drop completely down at the end of each repetition.

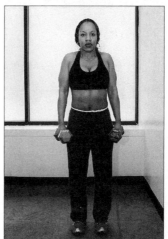

The Routine: The Basic Eight

Body Area: Triceps

■ Dumbbell Kickbacks

STARTING POSITION: In a lunge position, rest your left hand on your left thigh for support. Holding a dumbbell, bend your right arm and elevate your elbow.

THE MOVE: Keeping your upper arm pressed to your side with the elbow elevated, push the dumbbell up and out until your arm is fully extended. Return to the starting position in a controlled motion. Repeat with your left arm.

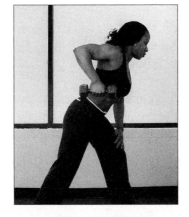

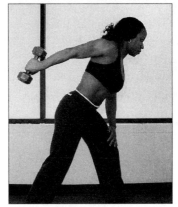

TRAINER'S TIPS

- Maintain proper spine and neck alignment.
- Keep your elbow elevated throughout the exercise.
- Focus your mind on your triceps.

The Routine: The Basic Eight

Body Area: Biceps

■ Standing Dumbbell Curls

STARTING POSITION: Stand with your feet shoulder-width apart, holding two dumbbells at your sides, palms facing in.

THE MOVE: Begin to curl both dumbbells simultaneously, rotating your palms as the weights pass your hips. Continue the smooth arc until the weights reach your shoulders. Then lower the dumbbells back to the starting position with your palms facing in.

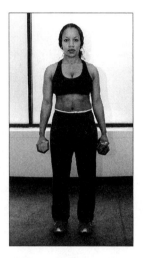

> **TRAINER'S TIPS**
>
> • Keep your upper arms motionless and pressed against your upper torso throughout the range of movement.
> • Aim for a smooth, flowing movement.
> • Focus your mind on your biceps.

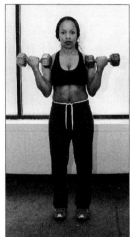

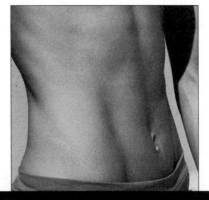

From Baby to Beach

by Debbie Holmes, M.S., Health and Exercise Education

*"From Baby to Beach" will guide you safely through the workout
basics during pregnancy and through the months that follow.*

CHAPTER ELEVEN

Abs and Babies

PREVIEW: *This chapter will guide you through your pregnancy from the perspective of training your abs.*

My Story

They always say you don't know what you're talking about until you've tried it. My experiences as a mother of three have taken me from a cesarean with my first baby to a traditional vaginal birth for my next two. As an exercise specialist, a health educator, and an owner of two training and rehab facilities, I make it my goal to work with most of the pregnant ladies who come through my gyms. Being pregnant is a positive, healthy, exciting, and dramatic time. It is also a unique time for each mom.

PREGNANCY ONE

The most frequent comment I received while pregnant with my first child was "Wow, you are going to have such an easy pregnancy." I guess people thought that since I worked out all day with my clients, I was bound to have an "easy" pregnancy. Well, it was mostly easy, until the last month. Because of complications, I had to have a cesarean. Fortunately, I understood how to get back to exercising without impeding the healing process.

PREGNANCIES TWO AND THREE

The amazing thing about getting pregnant with babies number two and three was that I knew more and so did my body. Have you ever heard of muscle memory? Well, when the hormones kicked in, the body knew it was time to prepare the womb again. This time, my abdominal muscles cooperated and all went well. This is where fitness helped me once again, because with my second and third pregnancies, I was able to deliver vaginally in a matter of a few hours. Lo and behold, it produced the same result.

Having experienced both types of deliveries, let me tell you why, barring complications, I feel that a natural, vaginal delivery is better. Your body recovers in half the time. You must take extra precautions while mending from a C-section. A cesarean section is a cut across the abdominal muscle wall; therefore the muscle fibers need to reattach and mend, which takes a little longer.

At our health and fitness clubs in Colorado, I help many of our members through this process. I'd like to help you on this journey, making your pregnancy—and return from pregnancy—a little easier.

To Train or Not to Train

One of the biggest misconceptions regarding pregnancy is that you need to quit doing abdominal exercises. Let me make one huge point: What muscles do you think you are going to use to push that kid out? Got it? That said, there are some serious precautions that need to be addressed. So let's talk about it.

How did exercise and abdominal exercises help me? Well, for my second and third kids, they gave me the ability to push effectively and focus on the proper muscles to use during childbirth. The process of giving birth is much like weight training. The breathing is controlled and focused. The pushing is direct and strong. If you learn the proper training techniques—how to control and focus your working muscles—and understand proper breathing, you won't waste strength and energy on useless pushes. Undirected and untrained pushes will only exhaust you more, making the whole experience harder.

Exercising also helps you develop the mind-muscle link. This connection will give you better control over your muscles. There are times during delivery when you need to relax, but your body is telling you to push. When you're in touch with your ab muscles, you can control them better. You can contract and relax them on command. Stronger muscles will respond to the stresses of pregnancy more effectively and efficiently than weak muscles.

Training your abs will also

- improve your endurance for labor
- strengthen your core stabilization muscles
- improve circulation in the ab area

As one of my friends told me, she loved doing her crunches because she felt like she was hugging her child each time she did one. Now you're training for love. But remember not to overdo it—just as you can overtrain when you're not pregnant, you can overtrain when you are, which could lead to complications.

The Three E's: Eating, Energy, and Exercise

The ideal pregnancy program would be a continuation of the program you are already on. However, pregnancy also motivates many people to start getting fit. That's great; yet let me warn you that it's the toughest time to start. As you know, your body will be experiencing changes unlike anything you've ever imagined. But don't let that stop you.

These changes happen before you even know that you are pregnant. It's because of those wonderful chemicals we call hormones. The minute you conceive, your body begins to release hormones that are associated with pregnancy. It's these hormones that cause sleepiness, fatigue, and nausea. These hormones prepare your body for the physical changes that are about to happen. The changes are usually most dramatic during your first trimester but will calm down as you enter your second trimester. Usually, the nausea will subside or ease up, allowing you the opportunity to eat.

EATING DURING PREGNANCY

Here's my opinion on eating more during pregnancy. Never let anyone convince you that you need to eat a lot more food when you are pregnant. Pregnancy is not an excuse to overeat. You should eat better, but simply increasing the quantity isn't the answer. This is why so many women get themselves into trouble by gaining too much weight during pregnancy. Remember, what you put on, you're going to want to take off.

During the first trimester, that little person inside of you is tiny and will not use up all the extra calories if you are overeating.

He or she is drawing nutrients from your normal diet. As the baby grows inside of you, the amount of calories he or she pulls from you will increase, but not in these early stages of pregnancy. So don't eat more, just eat better. As the baby grows, you'll need to adjust, with small increases.

Along with nausea, fatigue will be the other primary obstacle to overcome during your first trimester. I still remember how tired I got with my first pregnancy. I actually fell asleep in the middle of a mystery dinner party and missed the entire climax. It was uncontrollable at times. This is natural and expected, so don't get discouraged. Usually, this will pass and your energy will return somewhere around the second trimester. So, just how do you get that exercise session in when you are exhausted and have no energy?

Here's how I did it: I used to be a mid-afternoon exercise person. Not anymore. I had to move my exercise routine to the morning hours. It was the only time I had the energy. If I waited until the afternoon, I found myself taking a nap instead of working out. Hey, naps are important, so take them when you can . . . but remember to exercise. Fit exercise into your day when you have the time and energy.

Heart Rate

During pregnancy your heart rate increases fairly dramatically. Your heart is pumping faster at all hours of the day, and even harder during exercise. Remember that you are now pumping for two. The rule of thumb for pregnancy is to keep your heart rate under 140 beats per minute.

However, my experience has shown me that women who have exercised a long time prior to conceiving find it hard to keep under 140. You'll find that just walking around and up stairs will easily put you over that target. So for individuals who have a difficult time keeping their heart rate down, it's okay to work within the 140 to 160 heart-rate range. A good indicator is the speaking test. If you can carry on a conversation with someone next to you without losing your breath, that is a good indicator that you aren't overdoing it. A heart-rate monitor would be a good investment. You can wear it all the time. You'll be amazed at how high your heart rate goes during simple everyday tasks.

Heat

Even more important than your heart rate is your body temperature. Getting overheated is a definite no-no. Your baby can't cool itself off as quickly as you can. Heated conditions last longer in the womb. This can cause serious birth defects. You should never allow yourself to get really hot. That's why doctors do not want you to get into hot tubs. If you find yourself extremely hot, you'll need to cool off quickly. Once again, pay attention to what time of day you are exercising and where, and modify if you need to.

Relaxin

An important pregnancy hormone to be aware of is relaxin. Relaxin is released into your body in increasing amounts as you build toward your delivery. Relaxin softens and prepares your body for delivery. This is the reason that a child can be pushed through the pelvic cavity. This softening of the ligaments and joints will become more prevalent as you get closer to your delivery date. The truth is, you want it to peak right about delivery time. That way the baby comes out and your body can come back. It's an amazing cycle.

Relaxin isn't picky—all your joints and ligaments will be affected, so take caution with everything you do. Even basic stretching for all those aches and pains can become serious if done too hard. Do everything in moderation. Never overstretch any joint with relaxin moving through your body. You could seriously injure a joint, ligament, or tendon. With the relaxin in your body, it will also take an increased amount of time for those ligaments and tendons to heal. So pay attention to any activity that might cause unnecessary stress on your joints. You also need to be careful after delivery because relaxin remains in your body in decreasing amounts for up to one year after you have given birth.

Weight Training

This is a good time to mention precautions regarding weight training. You can keep up your normal routine throughout the first trimester and into the second. But lower your intensity. Don't push too hard. Your goal during pregnancy is to maintain, not make gains. Usually, somewhere around five or six months, you'll want to lower the amount of weight you're using and do more of a light toning workout. During those last few months, you need to stop any exercises that cause discomfort. Listen to your body. This is not the time to push through discomfort. Examples of exercises and equipment that you'll probably avoid during the third trimester are

- adduction (inner-thigh) movements
- leg presses and squats
- abdominal machines
- lower-back machines

It's okay to stop them for now; remember that you won't be pregnant forever.

Guidelines and Recommendations

The following are recommendations for exercise during pregnancy and postpartum by the American College of Obstetricians and Gynecologists. These guidelines are for women who do not have any risk factors for adverse maternal or perinatal outcomes.

1. During pregnancy, women can continue to exercise and derive health benefits from participating in mild- to moderate-intensity exercise routines.
2. Working heart rate should be measured during peak levels of activity to ensure that exercise intensity is within the desired range.
3. Regular exercise (at least three times per week) is preferable to intermittent activity.
4. Extremes of joint flexion and extension (such as deep knee bends and ballistic hyperextension of the knee) should be avoided.
5. Pregnant women should avoid exercising in the supine position (on their backs) after the first trimester.
6. Prolonged periods of motionless standing should be avoided.
7. Pregnant women should be aware of the decreased oxygen available for aerobic exercise and should be encouraged to modify exercise intensity according to maternal symptoms. Pregnant women should stop exercising when fatigued and not exercise to exhaustion.
8. Avoid exercises in which loss of balance could be detrimental to maternal or fetal well-being, especially in the third trimester. Any type of exercise involving the potential for even mild abdominal trauma should be avoided.
9. Women who exercise during pregnancy should be particularly careful to ensure an adequate diet.
10. Women should gradually increase exercise intensity after delivery.

In addition, women with certain other medical or obstetric conditions—including chronic hypertension and active thyroid, cardiac, vascular, or pulmonary disease—should be evaluated carefully in order to determine whether an exercise program is appropriate.

CHAPTER TWELVE

Exercising During Pregnancy

PREVIEW: *This chapter outlines a training routine for each trimester.*

Warning Signs

Because your body is experiencing so many changes, you need to pay extra attention to any signs of physical distress. If you experience any of the following, you need to stop the activity that you are doing and immediately call your doctor:

- spotting or bleeding
- cramping
- dizziness
- increased water retention
- sharp pains

- irregular heartbeat
- excessive soreness
- nausea and/or vomiting
- difficulty breathing
- excessive fatigue

Be Aware of the Round Ligament

Something that will increase near the end of your pregnancy is the sharp pain associated with the "round ligament" of the abdominal region. It will feel like someone has stabbed you in the stomach. That is the ligament literally being forced into a greater stretch. This pain will usually occur after a growth spurt and subside a little later in the day, only to occur again soon. I can always remember it grabbing me as I would get out of my car. That's when I knew baby and I had gotten a little bigger and it was time to loosen the maternity pants a little more.

Getting Ready to Train: Precautions

As I mentioned earlier, the abdominal muscles are going to help you deliver your child. So it is important to train them for the delivery. However, not everyone will have the ability to train while pregnant, so make sure you discuss everything with your physician.

Remember, it is not about how challenging the routine is, it's about keeping the abdominal muscles conditioned and becoming aware of how to push on demand.

You never want to push directly into your pelvic floor. This is different from a Kegel, where you lift or zip up the pelvic floor. Always think of raising the pelvic floor and not pushing down and out as if you were trying to push something out of your body. To get the feeling of what I am saying, try tightening your abdominals only; now try tightening your abdominals while pushing down into your pelvic floor. It's similar to the sensation you get when you are having a bowel movement. Remember this important tip throughout all your exercise training. Okay, let's train.

First Trimester

The Prescription: Do one set each of the following exercises and stay between ten and twenty repetitions, depending on your fitness level and how you are feeling during the workout. Do the routine three times a week.

Notes: You can also choose the butterfly position for crunches (page 39) if that is more comfortable. I know your body is going through a lot of changes; nevertheless, you need to be consistent. Try to follow through even if that means doing just five reps for each exercise.

EXERCISE	REPETITIONS	SETS	PEAK HOLD
Crunches: Knees Bent (page 188)	Between 10 and 20	1	1 second
Crossovers (page 172)	Between 10 and 20 on each side	1	1 second
Double Crunches (page 205)	Between 10 and 20	1	1 second
Basic Trunk Extensions (page 248)	Between 10 and 20	1	1 second

Second Trimester

As you start to grow and get bigger, you should limit how many exercises you do on your back. As the baby gets bigger, it presses down on major arteries. This inhibits the flow of blood from your extremities—primarily your legs—back to your heart. During this crucial period, the most important thing is to be safe.

The Prescription: Do one set each of the following exercises and stay between ten and twenty repetitions, depending on your fitness level and how you are feeling during the workout. Do the routine three times a week.

Notes: Remember the basic precautions: Keep your heart rate down and don't get overheated.

EXERCISE	REPETITIONS	SETS	PEAK HOLD
Pelvic Tilts (page 221)	Between 10 and 20	1	1 second
Side Bends with Weight (page 178)	Between 10 and 20 on each side	1	1 second
Crunches on Side (page 200)	Between 10 and 20 on each side	1	1 second
Tummy Tucks (page 224)	Between 10 and 20	1	1 second
Swimming on All Fours (page 250)	Between 10 and 20 on each side	1	1 second

The Third Trimester

Near the end of your pregnancy, because of the increased size of your belly, you might be able to perform just a couple of exercises. Remember to do only what is comfortable.

The Prescription: Do one set each of the following exercises and stay between ten and twenty repetitions, depending on your fitness level and how you are feeling during the workout. Do the routine three times a week.

Note: As your due date nears, your mind becomes more important. Since you don't want to push yourself too hard physically, you can up the commitment by really focusing on integrating your breathing with your muscle contraction while you exercise. This focus will help you when the big day comes.

EXERCISE	REPETITIONS	SETS	PEAK HOLD
Pelvic Tilts (page 221)	Between 10 and 20	1	1 second
Crunches on Side (page 200)	Between 10 and 20 on each side	1	1 second
Tummy Tucks (page 224)	Between 10 and 20	1	1 second
Swimming on All Fours (page 250)	Between 10 and 20 on each side	1	1 second

CHAPTER THIRTEEN

Getting Back in Bathing Suit Shape

PREVIEW: *This chapter takes you through the step-by-step process of getting back in shape.*

After the Baby Is Born: Common Questions

How is it that models get back in shape in only a few weeks?

Their return to normal is so abnormal. First, their business is their bodies. They are able to get themselves back in shape with the help and expense of many professionals, starting with personal trainers, cooks, nannies, and around-the-clock help. They are able to focus on their bodies 100 percent of the time. So you can't compare yourself to them.

Will nursing help me lose weight?

Another huge misconception is that you will lose weight while nursing. This may be true if you are nursing twins or triplets, but I never experienced weight loss while breast-feeding. You will lose some weight, but then the body still holds on to extra calories so that it can continue its production of breast milk. It wasn't until I stopped breast-feeding that those last ten pounds came off.

How soon can I start exercising?
Technically, some experts say you can start exercising twenty-four hours after giving birth. Are they crazy? I can't believe that anyone would have the energy or desire to do any kind of exercise outside of normal household activity. Exhaustion from the delivery, heavy bleeding, soreness, lack of sleep with a newborn, anxieties of motherhood, the hospital stay . . . do I need to go on? These are all reasons why your body is tired and needs rest. Rest allows the healing process to begin. So give yourself the time you need to heal.

What's a reasonable time frame?
Usually three to six weeks. It really depends on how you delivered and how you are healing. You should talk to your physician about getting your walking orders. By walking orders, I mean when the doctor says you can get out and walk for exercise. This means taking your baby out for a ten- or fifteen-minute walk. And it's always important to follow the signs that your body gives you: Has the bleeding stopped? Has the pain subsided? Have you gotten a few good hours of sleep? Once these kinds of signs start showing up in your life, then you can start getting back into your exercise routine.

When can I start my abdominal exercises?
As soon as you've been given the go-ahead from your physician. After a C-section, you need to watch movement that incorporates lower abdominal recruitment. The last thing you want to do is to tear open your scar, especially internally. After a C-section, you

will definitely need six weeks to recuperate. Then you should do only gentle, easy pelvic tilts and contractions until ten to twelve weeks. For a vaginal delivery, you'll be able to start back on a little quicker time frame.

You must understand that your abdominal muscles have been stretched and beaten up these last few months. With my third child, even seven months after delivery, my abs were still sore when I did my ab routine. This is normal and it is expected. So don't get discouraged; just do what you can do and then let them rest.

Will sex ever be the same again?
Absolutely! There are certain exercises (Kegels) that we will incorporate into your ab routine. Kegels will help prepare you for sex. The body is an amazing thing, and if you help it recover and heal properly, you will get back to normal in all activities. If you have any issues about resuming sexual intercourse, talk to your physician.

Will my incontinence subside?
This is true also for any bladder problems that might have been forced upon you during delivery. The Kegel exercises will help strengthen your entire pelvic floor, giving you benefits across the board. So plan on making the Kegels a part of your routine.

Is there any chance of getting my original body back?
Some women use the excuse of having children for their weight gain and they continue to use it the rest of their lives. It's only an excuse. Check out all those women in our everyday lives who are back to their slim, strong bodies. The key to getting your body back to its original weight is not to gain

more than you need to gain in the first place. I honestly believe that gaining more than a few pounds your first trimester is unnecessary. If you can keep the weight down the first trimester, then slowly put on weight starting at the end of the second trimester, you'll find yourself within the twenty-five to thirty pounds that defines the weight gain of a healthy pregnancy. Most of this comes off in short order—it's those last ten pounds that hang on, assuring good nutrition for nursing and healing. Don't get insane about taking it all off the day after delivery.

If you eat properly (for you and your baby), when you resume your exercise routine, your body will come back. When it does, treat yourself to a new outfit.

Kegels: Questioned Answers

What exactly is a Kegel?
Named after Dr. Arnold Kegel, Kegels strengthen the pubococcygeus (PC) muscle. This is the main muscle of the pelvic floor, which surrounds the vaginal, urethral, and rectal openings and is the major muscle of contraction during female orgasm. Strong pelvic muscles lend support, improve bladder control, increase sexual fulfillment, and can help rehabilitate some of the relaxation that may be caused by childbirth. By increasing blood supply to your pelvis, Kegels can also increase your resistance to urinary tract infections.

Where is my PC muscle?
To find your PC muscle, imagine that you're urinating and then stop the flow. You can also try this while you're really urinating, but it's not recommended to actually do a

series of Kegels then, because it can promote, rather than prevent, urinary tract infections.

How do I do Kegels?
Contract the PC muscle with a moderate, firm squeeze (about a 7 on a scale of 10), not a death grip. Hold the squeeze for ten seconds and then release. Do this ten times in a row, eventually working up to twenty-five in a row. For optimal results, experts recommend working up to seventy-five to eighty squeezes a day.

Make sure you are not contracting your ab, thigh, and butt muscles at the same time as your vaginal area. This will only increase intra-abdominal pressure, aggravating any existing urinary incontinence problem.

A TEST

To ensure that you are not contracting your abs at the same time that you contract your vaginal muscles, try this:

• Put two fingers in your vagina, spread apart slightly, and squeeze the vaginal muscles—you should feel these muscles tightening around your fingers. Put your other hand on your lower abdomen as a reminder to keep your belly soft and relaxed.

What can I expect?
To be effective, Kegels must be done correctly and regularly for at least three months before results can be expected. So take your time, and be patient and focus. Just as with crunches, these exercises work only when the right muscles are used, when the contraction is held long enough, and

when enough repetitions are done. To make Kegels a habit, try doing them

- while you watch TV
- before or after working out
- riding in a car or commuting to work
- at the movies
- at your desk at work

Getting Back in Shape: Rebuilding the Foundation

As mentioned earlier, your abdominal muscles will be sore for a while. They will work and function normally; however, they will get sore more easily. This is expected. These are growth pains as your muscles build back up to their normal size and strength. So you need to slowly return to your normal exercise routine.

STARTING THE PROGRAM

Vaginal Deliveries. You can start doing some basic easy exercises, like pelvic tilts, soon after delivery (only if you feel up to it). Three to four weeks is usually a safe time frame. When your physician gives you the go-ahead to start walking, then you should be able to begin Phase One of the program. This phase should usually last between three and six weeks. Remember, your abs may get sorer than normal and this will affect how hard you should push yourself. If

you're too sore to train for your next scheduled session, you did too much in your last session. Only move on to Phase Two when you feel you've built a foundation. This would mean you can do the routine without having to push yourself and you experience only mild soreness, if any at all.

C-Section Deliveries. C-section deliveries are much more invasive. You will not be able to engage in abdominal exercises for at least six weeks. You must get approval from your doctor. After all the healing has occurred, you can then begin with Phase One. Listen to your body, and if any of the exercises that follow elicit the feeling of pulling on your scar, *then back off that exercise until the skin has finished healing*. Stay with this phase for three to six weeks. Move on to Phase Two only when you've built a foundation. This would mean you can do the routine without having to push yourself and you experience only mild soreness, if any at all.

When you move on to Phase Two, also go slow and ease your body into the new routine.

Remember, if you experience any increased vaginal bleeding, bright red bleeding, pain, dizziness, or weakness, stop what you are doing and immediately contact your physician. You might be starting a little too soon. Rest, recover, and then try starting again in a week, with your physician's approval.

Phase One

GUIDELINES

Be gentle and go slow. If you have to rest at the bottom of the movement for a moment before you start your next repetition, that's fine. Take baby steps, giving yourself however much time you need to work up to twenty reps. If you need to rest between exercises, then rest. Before you move on to Phase Two, I want you to be able to complete the prescribed goals of this routine for three successive workouts.

The Prescription: Do this routine three times a week. The goal is to work up to twenty repetitions and to be able to do the entire routine without resting between exercises.

EXERCISE	REPETITIONS	SETS	PEAK HOLD
Pelvic Tilts (page 221)	20	1	1 second
Knee Raises (page 163)	20	1	1 second
Butterfly Crunches (page 190)	20	1	1 second
Catches (page 173)	20 on each side	1	1 second
Tummy Tucks (page 224)	20	1	1 second
Swimming on All Fours (page 250)	20	1	1 second

Phase Two: On the Road—Building Muscle and Endurance

GUIDELINES

Again, be gentle and go slow. If you have to rest at the bottom of the movement for a moment before you start your next repetition, that's fine. Take baby steps, giving yourself however much time you need to work up to twenty reps. If you need to rest between exercises, then rest. Before you move on to the System, I want you to be able to complete the prescribed goals of this routine for four successive workouts.

When you've completed Phase Two, you can start with Level One of the System. But follow the above guidelines for Phase One. Even though you've built a base, still err on the side of being careful. You'll have a moment, a click, when you know you're back for sure. Then you can start to push yourself harder.

The Prescription: Do this routine four times a week. The goal is to work up to twenty repetitions and to be able to do the entire routine without resting between exercises.

EXERCISE	REPETITIONS	SETS	PEAK HOLD
Reverse Crunches (page 160)	20	1	1 second
Double Crunches (page 205)	20	1	1 second
Catches (page 173)	10 on each side	1	1 second
Swimming on Belly (page 252)	20 on each side	1	1 second

Separation Anxiety

An abdominal complication from pregnancy is the separation of the abdominal wall down the middle of your stomach. It's called diastasis recti. You will know if this has occurred if there is a space directly down the middle of your stomach. The degree of separation can vary from one finger to many fingers. The greater the separation, the less chances you have to fix the problem on your own; it might require surgery after you've completed your family.

A GENTLE REMINDER

You can help the process by utilizing a technique that will help bring the separation together. As you do your ab exercises, simply pull your muscles toward the middle. It's not a strong pull, just a little pull in the right direction to focus your body and mind on your goal. The photos below illustrate a couple of ways to do the technique:

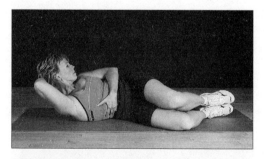

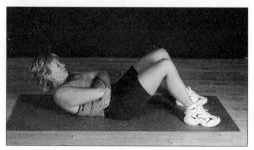

To Sum Up

You can get your old body back, even better than before, if the birth inspires you to new levels of fitness and wellness. The main thing is to be patient, to train your abs consistently, to do cardio work, ideally to start a basic weight-training program, and to eat intelligently. Also, use the power of your mind—really visualize the way you want your abs to look.

Now you have that deep motivation that was discussed in Chapter Seven, "The Mind." You're no longer exercising just for you. You need to stay strong and healthy for your child. You will also be teaching by example, showing your kid what a healthy lifestyle is.

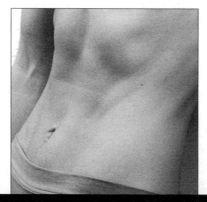

PART SIX

The Routines

*This part compiles routines to meet the training
needs of every stage of your life.*

CHAPTER FOURTEEN

Introduction to the Routines

PREVIEW: *This chapter shows you how to get the most out of the routines.*

Tips for Doing the Routines

The System and the routines in this book have done all the workout planning for you. The following guidelines will help you get the best results. One of the most important training principles is variety. You can't just stick with one routine forever. But you can always come back to a favorite routine after you've spent some time away. The important thing is to mix up your routines to keep your body and mind from getting bored. The routines in Chapter 15, "The Routines," will give you a variety of choices.

Chapter 16, "Creating Your Own Routine," will cover important principles for a lifetime of ab work.

MISSING WORKOUTS

Don't stress out if you miss a workout during the week; you haven't destroyed the whole program. Just get back in pace with the program. Remember, the key is consistency over the long haul. You can also double up on a day, doing two workouts back-to-back or one in the morning and one in the evening.

MAINTENANCE

The goal of any maintenance program is to keep the gains you've worked to achieve. Here are some tips for maintaining your gains and moving forward.

The System: To maintain the results of the System, stick with the program outlined in Level Three. Since it is easier to maintain than to build, you could even do each routine just once a week (the Traditional and the Functional) and maintain the majority of your gains. This won't work forever, but it could be a strategy to use for a four- to six-week period if you just don't have the time. Remember, the key is consistency over time.

There may be times when your schedule gets hectic and you do Level One or Level Two routines for a few weeks. Any of these choices will help you maintain the results you've worked to achieve. It's also a good way to create variety, so you don't get bored.

For a new challenge, you could also opt to do the Advanced Routine (page 135).

Sports Training: If you were doing one of the sports-specific routines on page 144 and the prescription was three times a week, you could reduce it to twice a week and maintain your strength gains. For example, let's say you were doing the Sports Challenge (page 144) and you started in the winter. Throughout the winter, you did it three times a week. Then spring rolls around, the weather starts to get warm, and you don't have as much time to work out, but you're using your core muscles doing your favorite sport. To maintain the benefits, do the routine once or twice a week. This will support your game and keep you from burning out on the routine.

You're like an athlete in season. Off-season, you did ab work for your sport. Now it's time to enjoy the game. But you don't want to lose all you worked for, so you have to put in some time to maintain it.

Substitution: If there is an exercise in a routine that you can't do for some reason—back pain, lack of equipment—then substitute it with an exercise that works the same area and has the same difficulty level. If it's an obliques exercise, go to Part Seven, "The Exercises," and pick one out. If you've exhausted all options, you can repeat an exercise that is already in the routine.

CHAPTER FIFTEEN

The Routines

PREVIEW: *This chapter outlines this roster of routines:*

The System— The Advanced Routine

This routine will challenge you with more-difficult exercises. As always, it is key to master the movements before pushing yourself too hard.

The Prescription: Do this routine three times a week. When you can comfortably reach the prescribed repetitions, increase the time you hold your peak contraction—up to three seconds. Increase the stakes by adding an-other set. Rest for two to three minutes; then perform the entire routine again. There is also a bonus add-on, if you are inspired.

■ Exercises

1. V-Ups with a Cross (page 214): Work up to 10 reps on each side.
2. Side Double Crunches (page 215): Work up to 15 reps on each side.
3. Superwomans with Rotation (page 255): Work up to 10 reps on each side.

4. Double Crunches with a Cross (page 206): Work up to 10 reps on each side.
5. Double Air Pumps (page 229): Work up to 15 reps.
6. Superwomans (page 253): Work up to 20 reps.
7. Corkscrews (page 162): Work up to 10 reps on each side.
8. Crunches with a Twist (page 207): Work up to 10 reps on each side.
9. Swimming on Belly (page 252): Work up to 10 reps on each side.

Bonus Exercises for the Driven

10. Reverse Crunches (page 160): Work up to 15 reps.
11. Butterfly Crunches (page 190): Work up to 15 reps.
12. Basic Trunk Extensions (page 248): Work up to 15 reps.

Ab Asanas (Postures)

In Sanskrit, *yoga* means "union," a joining together. The root word in Sanskrit means "to yoke." Yoga is about connecting your mind, body, and spirit. The following quick overview will outline some key yoga principles to integrate into your workout.

BASIC PRINCIPLES

1. Start each session with a brief relaxation to center your mind and accept how your body feels in the moment. Every day you're living in a new body.
2. Breathe evenly through your nose during the posture. Breath, or *prana*, is the energy of life, the energy of the universe. When you breathe fully, you hook into the powerful energy grid of the universe. The breath is the energy that supports the movement from the inside, energizing and empowering your muscles.
3. Stay tuned in. Remain present and stay focused on your breath and the posture. Your breath and the posture will teach you about your mind and your body.
4. Be aware of your alignment. During the plank movements, make sure your entire body stays in a straight alignment: ankles with knees, knees with hips, hips with shoulders, shoulders with ears.
5. Integrate knowledge into action. This means that you should stay open to the feedback your awareness is giving you and adjust. Everyone will need to make different adjustments—lowering hips, keeping the breath steady, and even bringing one's mind back to the task. Integration and awareness are at the heart of what yoga means, yoking and joining together the elements of mind, body, and breath into a flowing, dancelike, seamless whole.

Yoga is about fostering a good attitude. This is one of the major differences in its approach to exercise. Part of the practice is bringing your mind to the workout with a positive attitude. In the West, exercise is often thought of as an evil we must endure. We hate it, even as we force ourselves to do it.

Yoga attempts to bring our mind/attitude into a healthier relationship with exercise. In the West, when it comes to exercise, the end often justifies the means—grin and bear it. Yoga asks you to bring a mindfulness to the task. After all, part of the goal of living is to find love and joy in the things that are difficult and challenge us.

One way to do this is to apply the above principles each time you work out. You need to apply these principles to all your workouts: lifting, cardio, and traditional ab work. This is one of the great lessons yoga can teach.

George Feuerstein, a leading yoga teacher and practitioner, says, "Yoga is first and foremost the discipline of conscious living." Awareness is the umbrella that covers all these basic principles.

THE ROUTINES

The following routines take moves from hatha yoga. Since yoga has entered the mainstream, these moves are also done in many non-yoga exercise classes.

Routine One: Plank Flow

The Prescription: Work up to holding the down plank and each side plank for thirty seconds. Start out with a ten-second hold and increase in five-second intervals, as you are ready.

■ Exercises

1. Down Plank (page 257)
2. Side Plank (page 257)

Yoga Variation: Move from the down plank to a side plank, rotating onto your left arm, raising your right arm, and holding for the prescribed time. Then move back through the down plank, just pausing for a moment, and into another side plank, rotating on your right arm, raising your left arm, and holding for the prescribed time.

Routine Two: Power Moves

The Prescription: Work up to the recommended repetitions at your own pace.

■ Exercises

1. Reverse Superwomans (page 254)
2. Leg-Overs: Double Leg (page 183)

REVERSE SUPERWOMANS: Hold the movement for 10 seconds, then lower. Work up to 5 repetitions on each side.

LEG-OVERS: DOUBLE LEG: Keep the movement slow and controlled—5 seconds to lower the legs and 5 seconds to raise them back to the starting position. Repeat to the other side with the same five-count. Work up to 5 repetitions on each side without resting between reps.

Pilates: Sequencing the Spine

WHAT IS PILATES?

Though it may appear to be the latest fitness craze, Pilates was actually developed in Germany in the late 1800s by Joseph Pilates. He designed a unique combination of stretching and strengthening exercises that condition every part of the body, increase circulation and cardiovascular strength, and rid the body of toxins. Precision is the key element in reaping the benefits from the Pilates system. This means learning the basic terms and techniques used to direct proper execution of the movements.

Powerhouse. Pilates uses this term to describe the band of muscles that circles your body from just below the bottom of your ribs to just below your butt. This is roughly the same area that's now referred to as the core. It includes your abdominal, lower-back, hip, and buttock muscles. In Pilates, this also includes the deep inner muscles—the transverse abdominis and the pelvic floor. In Pilates, all exercises are initiated from this powerhouse area. To properly utilize the powerhouse, you need to engage these muscles and lengthen the space between the bottom of your ribs and the tops of your hips.

"Scooping" Your Belly. This movement, along with contracting your buttocks, will help stabilize and anchor your body. Scooping does not mean sucking in your belly and holding your breath. You use your transverse abdominis muscle to scoop your belly in while the rest of your body, including your breath, moves freely. Imagine your belly button is actually drawn toward your spine by a magnetic force.

Pilates Leg/Foot Position: Also called the "Pilates stance," this involves the whole leg, from hip to heel. When your legs are straight, squeeze your heels together and turn your toes out in a small V while rotating your thighs away from each other. This engages the backs of your legs and your buttocks and stabilizes your hips as an anchor point. Again, imagine that your legs are being pulled together by a magnetic force from the inside of your heels to the tops of your inner thighs.

Let's take a look at how the above techniques work in the context of the classic Pilates move the roll-up. Pilates involves more than this short introduction. To get a full sense of the system, you should buy a book specializing in Pilates, try one of the Pilates tapes, or take a class with a qualified instructor.

The Prescription: Complete ten roll-ups. Work up to this goal gradually. The most important thing is quality, not quantity. Follow the training tips and Pilates principles outlined.

■ Roll-Ups *(page 226)*

TRAINER'S TIPS

- Peel your spine off the mat one vertebra at a time. This begins with your neck. Reverse the order on the way back down, starting with the lowest vertebra of your spine.
- Keep your abdomen scooped in for the entire movement.
- Don't let your spine bulge out as you execute the movement.
- Maintain a Pilates leg/foot position.
- Let your breath fill your rib cage as you keep your inner core activated.
- Keep the exercise precise and moving with a steady flow.

The Office Routine
by Mike Brungardt

This routine is designed to give you an ab workout without your ever having to leave your office chair. You can do it during a break, right before lunch, or at the end of the day. It's also a fun way to work off a little stress. The routine has three levels. Stay with each level for at least two weeks before moving on.

KNEE RAISES: From a seated position, raise both knees toward your chest. Work up to 20 reps.

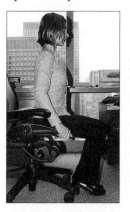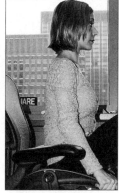

DOUBLE CROSSES: Cross your opposite shoulder and knee toward each other. Work up to 20 reps.

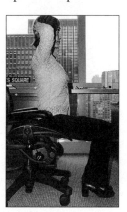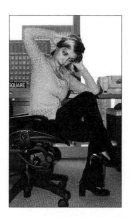

TRUNK EXTENSIONS: Place your hands behind your head, bend at the waist, and lower your chest toward your knees. Then use your lower-back muscles to raise your torso back to the starting position. Work up to 20 reps.

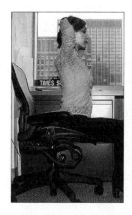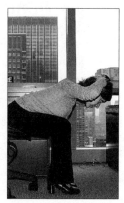

The Body Bar Routine
by Martin Kammler

The body bar is an easy and safe way to add resistance to your ab routine. The following exercises will introduce you to the basics, then you can get creative.

THE PRESCRIPTION

BODY BAR CRUNCHES: KNEES BENT: Work up to 20 reps.

BODY BAR CATCHES: Work up to 20 reps on each side.

BODY BAR REVERSE CRUNCHES: Work up to 20 reps.

PUSH CRUNCHES: Work up to 20 reps.

■ Body Bar Crunches: Knees Bent

DIFFICULTY: 1
LOWER BACK: LOW RISK
AREA OF FOCUS: UPPER ABS

STARTING POSITION: Lie flat on your back with your knees bent and both feet on the floor. Place the body bar between your legs and hold it in front of your chest, one hand on top of the other.

THE MOVE: Use your upper abs to raise your shoulder blades off the floor in a forward curling motion, moving the body bar with you. When you reach the top of the movement, extend your arms, pushing the body bar away from your body. Then lower your torso back to the starting position. Repeat the movement. Work up to 20 reps.

TRAINER'S TIPS

• Keep constant tension on your abs throughout the movement.
• Focus your mind on feeling your upper abs do the work.
• Don't rest at the bottom of the movement.
• Hold the contraction at the top of the movement.
• Keep a neutral spine.
• Alternate your grip on the way down, changing the bottom hand to the top.

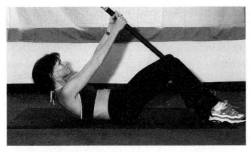

VARIATIONS: You can do many of the crunch variations in Part Seven, "The Exercises," in the same way.

■ Body Bar Catches

DIFFICULTY: 2
LOWER BACK: LOW RISK
AREA OF FOCUS: OBLIQUES

STARTING POSITION: Lie flat on your back with your knees bent and both feet on the floor. Place the body bar outside your left leg, holding it with one hand on top of the other, like an oar.

THE MOVE: Use your ab muscles to raise your torso diagonally, pushing the body bar up and out at an angle as your hands move outside and above your left knee. Then, in a controlled motion, lower your torso back to the floor. Repeat the movement to the opposite side. Work up to 20 reps on each side.

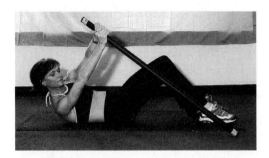

TRAINER'S TIPS

- Make sure you get both arms outside the knee and slightly above knee level.
- Keep your lower back supported on the floor.
- Focus your mind on your oblique muscles as you cross from side to side.
- Alternate your grip on the way down, changing the bottom hand to the top.

■ Body Bar Reverse Crunches

DIFFICULTY: 2
LOWER BACK: LOW RISK
AREA OF FOCUS: LOWER ABS

STARTING POSITION: Lie flat on your back; raise your thighs so your knees are above your hips with your lower legs (calves and feet) parallel to the floor. Position the body bar just below your knees and gently hold it in place with your hands.

THE MOVE: Focusing on your lower abs, curl your hips off the floor toward your rib cage, moving your knees toward your forehead so your hips come off the floor two to three inches. Hold the contraction at the top of the movement. Then lower your hips in a controlled motion, keeping tension on your abs. As your hips touch the floor, repeat the movement. Work up to 20 reps.

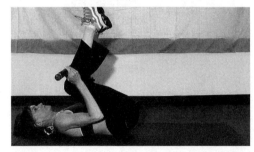

TRAINER'S TIPS

- Make sure your abs are doing the work. Don't rock, using momentum.
- Don't rest your hips on the floor at the end of the movement.
- Keep constant tension on your abs.
- Focus your mind on your lower abs.

■ Push Crunches

DIFFICULTY: 2
LOWER BACK: LOW RISK
AREA OF FOCUS: UPPER ABS

STARTING POSITION: Lie flat on your back with your knees bent and both feet on the floor. Hold the bar directly above your shoulders, arms extended.

THE MOVE: Use your upper abs to raise your shoulder blades off the floor, as if you were pushing the bar straight up instead of curling forward. Lower your shoulders back to the starting position and repeat the movement. Work up to 20 reps.

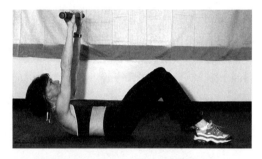

TRAINER'S TIPS

- Keep constant tension on your abs throughout the movement.
- Focus your mind on feeling your upper abs do the work.
- Don't rest at the bottom of the movement.
- Hold the contraction at the top of the movement for a count of two.
- Keep your neck lengthened.
- Keep a neutral spine.

The California Circuit
by Steven Wilde

This is a quick workout that trains your entire abdominal area and your lower back. For an extra challenge, repeat the circuit. You don't need to rest between circuits, because your abs get a break during your lower-back work.

The Prescription: To execute this routine, begin by crossing your left leg in the figure 4 position. Do a set of crunches, followed by crossovers, bringing your right shoulder toward your left knee. Then finish with reverse crunches. Complete this sequence with no rest between exercises. You're not done yet. Roll over on your belly for a set of Superwomans.

■ Exercises

1. Crunches: Figure 4 (page 198) 20 reps
2. Crossovers (page 172) 20 reps on each side
3. Reverse Crunches (page 160) 20 reps (Repeat, switching the figure 4 position to the other leg.)
4. Superwomans (page 253) 20 reps

Gym Superset
by Dave Johnson

This is a quick gym routine using weight. Since these are supersets, you don't rest between exercises The goal is to add a little size to your abs so your cuts are more noticeable. The routine has two parts. Part One is for your abs. Part Two is for your lower back. This way, you build strength 360 degrees around your body.

GUIDELINES

- Complete this routine three times a week.
- Perform all of your sets in Part One, then complete your sets for Part Two.
- Do both exercises without resting, then take a two-minute break and repeat the sequence for a second set. Work up to three sets.

PART ONE: ABS

HANGING KNEE RAISES WITH A CROSS
(page 218): Hold a dumbbell between your feet. Use a weight that will allow you to do between 8 and 12 reps. When you can do 12 reps, add weight.

CABLE CRUNCHES WITH A CROSS
(page 220): Keep your reps between 8 and 12. When you can do 12 reps, add weight.

PART TWO: LOWER BACK

BACK EXTENSION: ROMAN CHAIR
(page 265): Secure your feet under the supports, then a weight plate to your chest. Use a weight that will allow you to do between 8 and 12 reps. When you can do 12 reps, add weight.

ON THE BALL: TORSO CORKSCREWS
(page 245): Hold a weight plate to your chest with one hand. Use a weight that will allow you to do between 8 and 12 reps. When you can do 12 reps, add weight.

Teen Routine

Working out should be fun and a challenge. All the exercises in this routine give you a clear goal. You reach for your knees, heels, and ankles. When you've mastered this routine, move on to Level One of the System.

The Prescription: Work up to thirty reps for all three exercises.

■ Exercises

1. Knee Touches (page 199)
2. Heel Touches (page 185)
3. Ankle Reaches (page 263)

Kid Fit

This routine is for the preteen. Its goal is to build strength and coordination in a fun and imaginative way.

The Prescription: Become the inchworm and try to do ten reps in a row as you move across the living room. Get your mom and dad to do it. It's not just for kids.

■ Inchworm *(page 262)*

The Sports Challenge

The sports routine is designed to train your body from a variety of angles, making your entire center stable and strong. It will give your abs and core an athletic base to improve performance and prevent injury. Make sure you have a good base of strength before you do this routine. A good preparation would be to work your way through the System.

The Prescription: Do the entire routine without resting between exercises.

■ Exercises

1. Leg Raises: Circles (page 168):
   Work up to 10 reps in each direction.
2. Crunch Circles (page 203):
   Work up to 10 reps in each direction.
3. Superwomans with Rotation (page 255):
   Work up to 10 reps on each side.
4. Roll-Ups (page 226):
   Work up to 20 reps.
5. Plank: Swimming (page 258):
   Work up to 10 reps on each side.
6. Plank: Swinging Gate (page 259):
   Work up to 10 reps on each side.
7. Plank: Flutters (page 260):
   Work up to 10 reps on each side.
8. V-Ups with a Cross (page 214):
   Work up to 10 reps on each side.
9. Low Twists (page 227):
   Work up to 10 reps on each side.
10. Sun Salutations (page 261):
    Work up to 10 reps on each side.

The Time Routines: One-, Two-, and Three-Minute Workouts
by Brett Brungardt

These routines will give you a quick ab workout when time is of the essence. One minute during a commercial break is better than nothing.

ONE-MINUTE ONE-EXERCISE WONDER

This exercise will work your entire abdominal area.

DOUBLE CRUNCHES WITH A CROSS *(page 206)*: Work up to 10 reps on each side.

TWO-MINUTE ROUTINE

■ Exercises

1. Corkscrews (page 162):
   Work up to 10 reps on each side.
2. Crunches with a Twist (page 207):
   Work up to 10 reps on each side.

THREE-MINUTE ROUTINE

■ Exercises

1. Hip-Ups (page 16):
   Work up to 20 reps.
2. Toe Touches with a Twist (page 209):
   Work up to 10 reps on each side.
3. Double Crunches (page 205):
   Work up to 20 reps.
4. Superwomans with Rotation (page 255):
   Work up to 10 reps on each side.

Senior Abs
by Debbie Holmes

ABDOMINAL CONCERNS FOR THE FIFTY-PLUS GANG

In most cases, there are very limited concerns you need to be aware of.

When doing ab work, you need to refrain from exercises that do not support the lower back and exercises that put undue stress on the hips, elbows, or shoulders.

In order to assure safety for your older age group, it may be advisable to concentrate on duration of exercise instead of intensity. You should increase the number of repetitions instead of increasing the difficulty levels of the exercises. The exercises in this routine will be safe and effective.

■ Crunches: Knees Up *(page 189)*

Beginners: 10 to 20 reps
Intermediate: 20 to 40 reps
Advanced: Up to 50 reps

■ Crossovers *(page 172)*

Beginners: 5 to 10 reps on each side
Intermediate: 10 to 20 reps on each side
Advanced: Up to 25 reps on each side

■ Reverse Crunches *(page 160)*

Beginners: 5 to 10 reps
Intermediate: 15 to 20 reps
Advanced: Up to 25 reps

■ Basic Trunk Extensions
(page 248)

Beginner: 10 to 20 reps
Intermediate and advanced: Up to
    40 reps

On the Slant

A slant board uses gravity to add resistance. This routine takes advantage of gravity from two different angles, giving you a simple and intense workout by alternating the two exercises. Most slant boards are adjustable, so increase the angle as you get stronger.

GUIDELINES
- Do not rest between exercises or sets unless needed.
- Increase repetitions as needed, maintaining the five-rep intervals.
- You can add weight to the exercises to stay within the repetition guidelines.

■ Exercises

FIRST SET

1. Reverse Crunches (page 160): 20 reps (head at the top of the board)
2. Crunches (page 188): 20 reps on each side (head at the bottom of the board)

SECOND SET

1. Reverse Crunches: 15 reps
2. Crunches: 15 reps on each side

THIRD SET

1. Reverse Crunches: 10 reps
2. Crunches: 10 reps on each side

Twenty-Something Breakdowns

This routine attacks the abs from opposite ends while also targeting the lower and upper obliques. This routine is designed for the advanced exerciser.

GUIDELINES

- Do not rest between exercises unless needed.
- Keep rest time between sets to a minimum (under thirty seconds).
- Eventually, do the entire routine without resting.

■ Exercises

FIRST SET

1. Corkscrews (page 162): 10 reps on each side
2. Crunches: Legs Straight Out (page 192): 21 reps

SECOND SET

1. Corkscrews: 8 reps on each side
2. Crunches: Legs Straight Out: 16 reps

THIRD SET

1. Corkscrews: 7 reps on each side
2. Crunches: Legs Straight Out: 14 reps

FOURTH SET

1. Corkscrews: 6 reps on each side
2. Crunches: Legs Straight Out: 12 reps

FIFTH SET

1. Corkscrews: 4 reps on each side
2. Crunches: Legs Straight Out: 8 reps

SIXTH SET

1. Corkscrews: 2 reps on each side
2. Crunches: Legs Straight Out: 4 reps

SEVENTH SET

1. Corkscrews: 1 rep on each side
2. Crunches: Legs Straight Out: 2 reps

Lower-Back System

This is a multilevel routine for your lower back. It is designed to be flexible and progressive. It is a good routine to combine with your ab work.

The Prescription: Stay with each level until you can do the prescribed number of repetitions, without resting between exercises, for three consecutive workouts.

Doing this routine twice a week will maintain your benefits. You can stop at any level that is appropriate for your fitness level.

■ Exercises

LEVEL ONE: This routine is designed for the beginner. Stay with this level until you can do the prescribed number of repetitions, without resting between exercises, for three consecutive workouts.

1. Pelvic Rock (page 222): 10 rocks (back and forth equals one rock)
2. Pelvic Clock (page 223): 3 in each direction

3. Down Cat—Up Cat (page 98): 5 repetitions
4. Swimming on All Fours (page 250): 15 reps on each side

LEVEL TWO: At Level Two, continue to do all the Level One exercises. Stay at this level until you can do the prescribed number of repetitions, without resting between exercises, for three consecutive workouts.

1. Basic Trunk Extensions (page 248): 20 reps
2. Swimming on Belly (page 252): 15 reps on each side

LEVEL THREE: At Level Three, continue to do all the Level One and Level Two exercises until you can do the prescribed number of repetitions for all three levels, without resting between exercises, for three consecutive workouts.

1. Superwomans (page 253): 15 reps
2. Superwomans with Rotation (page 255): 10 reps on each side

CHAPTER SIXTEEN

Creating Your Own Routine

PREVIEW: *This chapter will give you the tools you need to design your own routine so you can become your own personal trainer.*

The Design Model

When creating an ab routine, you need a basic design model or blueprint to work from. You can think of the abs as four separate boxes that comprise three areas: lower abs (Area One), obliques (Area Two), and upper abs (Area Three). You also need to include at least one lower-back exercise in your routine.

To build a routine, you need to think about how you want to shape and strengthen each area or box. This will depend on your individual needs and goals: weak areas, the look you want, sports-specific training. It is always important, however, to keep muscle balance in mind.

Since the exercises in this book are categorized according to the three basic ab areas, you'll find it easy to plug in exercises and personalize your routine.

Basic Concepts

The following are key principles (along with the principles in Chapter Two, "Ab Basics") you need to consider when building your routine.

MUSCLE BALANCE

The exercises you choose should work all the muscle groups in the abdominal area (see "Your Exercise Anatomy," page 11) at a variety of angles.

Never completely neglect one abdominal area to work weaker areas. If you have strong areas, still train them, but not as intensely as the weak areas. This means choosing exercises of less intensity, doing fewer reps, using fewer exercises for those areas, or any combination of the above.

Muscle balance is a key consideration when choosing exercises. The abdominal muscles work together during most activities. They also play an important role in supportive and structural alignment. When one muscle or muscle group becomes considerably stronger than another, the potential for injury is greatly increased.

EXERCISE ORDER

In general, the best order for exercises is from largest muscles to smallest. But the order can also be affected by individual goals and the need for variety. If your primary goal is to shape your obliques, then you will want to target them first. But staying with the same exercise order for extended periods of time will cause complacency (no adaptation), which means less-than-optimal gains.

VOLUME

Volume as it relates to abdominal strength training can be described as the total number of repetitions and the number of sessions per day, week, month. When creating a progressive series of routines, you want to keep an eye on total volume, making sure you're doing enough but not too much. Volume also relates to the intensity. of the exercises. When intensity increases, volume should decrease.

INTENSITY

Intensity relates to the difficulty of an exercise, the amount of resistance (weight), if any, and the amount of rest time.

VARIATION

Variation is the most neglected training principle. Training needs to be varied for the following reasons: to prevent overtraining, to avoid training plateaus, and to alleviate the boredom of monotonous training.

Variation is related to intensity and volume. When you first start working your abs, it is easier to shock your muscles and cause adaptation. As you become more advanced, you need to change your workouts more frequently. An example of how to do this is to choose exercises of greater difficulty that will naturally decrease your repetitions (volume) while increasing your intensity. Another way to create variety is to do the opposite: Increase your repetitions and decrease your intensity. When you're considering variations in volume and intensity, you may want to vary similar training days within a training week. You will have a day of high-intensity training (heavy) and one of low-intensity training (light). The terms *heavy* and *light* can be misnomers. To obtain the optimal training effect, overload (i.e., muscle failure) should always occur— on both "heavy" and "light" days.

Periodization

Periodization is a systematic and progressive training method designed to aid in planning and organization. This cyclical training encompasses all the basic training principles and helps bring performance to a peak. It is utilized by the greatest athletes and strength coaches in the world (many of whom have contributed to this book).

The scope of this book does not allow for a detailed treatment of periodization, but the following summary will help you in creating your abdominal routines. The basis for periodization was the General Adaptation Syndrome (GAS), developed during the 1930s. It was intended to describe a person's ability to adapt to stress. According to GAS, there are three distinct phases of adaptation:

1. *The alarm stage:* This relates to the individual's initial response to training. This could result in a temporary drop in performance due to stiffness and soreness.
2. *The resistance stage:* This is when the exerciser adapts to the training stimulus by making gains in strength, tone, and endurance.
3. *The overtraining stage:* If the stress placed upon the exerciser is too great, then the following can happen:

- plateauing and a decreased performance level
- chronic fatigue
- loss of appetite
- loss of body weight, or lean body mass
- increased illness potential
- increased injury potential
- decreased motivation and low self-esteem

During this stage, the desired training adaptations are not likely to occur. Outside stresses—for example, social life, nutrition, amount of sleep, work—also need to be considered to avoid overtraining.

The goal, then, is to remain in the resistance stage of training, where your body is making the compensations to the stresses applied and continually improving. This is where the concepts of periodization apply.

THE CYCLES

Once your goals have been defined, the next step is planning, which can be divided into four training phases. Before going into these cycles, you will need a definition of the peaking period, which is the goal of all these cycles.

The Peaking Period

This is the period where all of your training culminates, bringing out the best possible results. This will, of course, be different for everybody, depending on individual goals. For the elite athlete, this can be very complicated, because several variables have to come together at once: strength, endurance, sports-specific skill, diet, mental state. The same is true for a bodybuilder. Things become simplified if it's just the stomach you're concerned about. But even then, things aren't that simple. If you want your abs to peak out for a vacation on the beach, you should be focusing on three variables: your ab routine, your diet, and cardiovascular work. Again, the peaking period is when you bring all these elements together at their highest level.

Macrocycle

The macrocycle is the longest of the training phases. Its length varies from one individual to another, depending on the goals.

In general, the macrocycle lasts from the end of one peaking period to the beginning of the next peaking period. The macrocycle defines long-term goals and a specific time frame in which you want to peak: six weeks, six months, one year. The macrocycle contains three components: preparation (mesocycles and microcycles), peaking, and transition.

Mesocycle
The next-longest phase is the mesocycle. Mesocycles make up a macrocycle. The number, length, and purpose of your mesocycles will depend on the goals of your macrocycle. A mesocycle is a phase that has specific goals. For example, the goal of the first mesocycle may be that of preparation, which might include high-volume and fairly low-intensity training to build a base of strength. The next mesocycle's goals might include an increase in intensity (more difficult exercises, shorter rest periods) while maintaining volume requirements to build strength and endurance.

The next mesocycle goals may be oriented for strength gains (increase in intensity; increase in resistance, sets, or rest time; lower volume). The final mesocycle, in which you reach peak condition, might include more intensive evaluation: What areas are weak and need extra work; what areas are strong; what has worked best in the past; diet, mental state? Peaking for abdominals will differ from peaking for sports performance. Training intensity and volume may continue to increase when you're bringing your abs to a peak. When peaking for sports performance, they decrease, allowing for rest and recuperation before the event. The better the prepara-

tion—that is, the better your condition—the longer you will be able to maintain your peak.

Microcycle
Within each mesocycle are smaller units called "microcycles." Microcycles further refine the objectives by manipulating training variables on a daily basis. One day might include training of high volume (reps) and moderate intensity, while the next day may include training of high intensity and moderate volume (reps).

Transition
Unfortunately, maintaining peak anything for a long period of time can be very difficult. The cycle following a peaking period is the transition phase. The abdominals can maintain a peak longer than most muscle groups. So the possibility exists when training the abs to have more frequent and longer peaking periods. This is not to say that your abs can't look great all the time. And the concepts of the transition phase will help ensure this.

A transition phase allows for regeneration and recuperation, both mentally and physically. It also introduces variety into the program. The transition phase allows you to start at a higher training level in the next macrocycle. Without a transition phase, the rigors of peaking will ultimately lead us into stage three of the GAS: overtraining. The body needs time off from the peaking phase, with its diet restrictions and the high intensity of training. The transition phase allows the right amount of recovery so you jump right back to a growth phase.

When most people think of recuperation, they think of sitting on their butts and doing nothing. With the transition phase, this is not true. You continue to train but at lower volumes and intensities. Substitute activities you like. Have fun! Do light abdominal work once or twice a week. No more than sixty repetitions per day should be undertaken.

Using the design model at the beginning of this chapter and following the principles outlined in Chapter Two, "Ab Basics," you can choose exercises from this book to match the different ab areas and create your own customized routine. Then, following the natural cycles of periodization, you can create a series of progressive routines, staying as long as possible in the growth and peaking phases, to achieve the abs you want.

A CASE STUDY:
GETTING READY FOR THE BEACH

For example, if you wanted to peak for a vacation in Hawaii during the first week of March and it is now the beginning of December, you would plan a three-month macrocycle.

You would probably want to break this down into one-month mesocycles with two-week microcyles for the first two months and one-week microcycles for the last month, as you prepare to peak.

Your breakdown may go something like this:

First month: This would be your prepara-tion period. You would build a safe foundation doing low-intensity exercises with high reps. During your two microcycles, you would gradually decrease your rest time.

Second month: During this period, you would add exercises and increase the intensity of your workout. You would use your two-week microcycles to accomplish these goals. The goal of the first microcycle would be to add one new exercise per area. In the second microcycle, you would replace certain exercises with more difficult ones.

Third month: During this cycle, you would start to change your workouts more often, going to one-week microcycles. You may have a heavy week, adding isometric holds, followed by a week of high repetitions with no rest between sets. This could be followed by a week where you mix your light and heavy days. And during the last microcycle, you would train every day in preparation for peaking out for that first day on the beach. During this week, you may train more instinctively, switching your workout every day and training weak areas.

Also, during this week, all other facets of your training must peak (diet, cardiovascular exercise, and strength training).

Good luck with your advanced principles. The application of these principles will lead to your ultimate success and longevity in training.

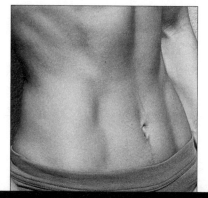

PART SEVEN

The Exercises

In this part you learn how to do the exercises safely and effectively.

CHAPTER SEVENTEEN

Introduction to the Exercises

PREVIEW: *This chapter explains the different elements in the exercise descriptions.*

The Exercises: A Method to the Madness

There are hundreds of ab exercises and variations. I know it can be overwhelming. The goal of this book is to give you a range of choices so you can always have variety in your workouts. At the same time, I want this selection to be ordered and easy to use. Below are explanations of the guidelines.

These guidelines are not objective standards that will be true for everyone. Certain movements are going to be easy or difficult, low or high risk, depending on your per-

sonal history. But the guidelines can be a helpful starting place.

Difficulty. This gives you guidance on how difficult the exercise is—1 being the easiest and 3 being the hardest. If you've been training consistently for a year and have a strong and healthy lower back, you should be able to do most of the exercises in this book. Some, obviously, will present more of a challenge. Safety must always come first. If you are unsure, consult a qualified professional.

Lower Back. This gives you guidance on the risk of injury to the lower back—low, moderate, or high. You need to be especially careful of your lower back. If you have a history of lower-back problems, you need to proceed with extra care and consult a specialist for advice on your specific condition.

Area of Focus. This tells you which body area you are training—lower abs, upper abs, obliques, lower back. Exercises that work more than one area are grouped together as combo movements.

Starting Position. This explains the proper starting position.

The Move. This outlines correct movement for the exercise.

Trainer's Tips. This acts as a personal trainer, giving you exercise tips. Some of the tips will be specific to the exercise. Others will be constant reminders, tips that are true for every exercise. Like hearing the inspiring voice of your personal trainer at your side, hearing these tips over and over may get annoying, but hearing them repeatedly will make them second nature. The following tips are essential for ab work:

1. Activate your inner core.
2. Keep constant tension on your abs.
3. Keep the motion controlled, for both the positive and the negative phases of the movement—no bouncing or jerking.
4. Pause for the contraction at the top of the movement.
5. Don't rest at the beginning of each new repetition before you begin the next one. Don't give your body weight to the floor. Let your shoulder blades or hips just lightly touch.
6. Focus your mind on feeling your abs do the work. Put your mind in the muscle—don't just go through the motions.
7. Keep your neck lengthened and have the proper spacing between your chin and your chest—apple- or fist-distance.
8. Breathe!

CHAPTER EIGHTEEN

Area One: Lower Abs

PREVIEW: *This chapter introduces exercises that train your lower abs.*

■ ■ ■

■ Reverse Crunches

DIFFICULTY: 2
LOWER BACK: LOW RISK
AREA OF FOCUS: LOWER ABS

STARTING POSITION: Lie flat on your back; raise your thighs so your knees are above your hips, placing your lower legs (calves and feet) parallel to the floor. You can place your hands either at your sides or behind your head.

THE MOVE: Focusing on your lower abs, curl your hips off the floor toward your rib cage, moving your knees toward your forehead so your hips come off the ground two to three inches. Hold the contraction at the top of the movement. Then lower your hips in a controlled motion, keeping tension on your abs. As your hips touch the floor, repeat the movement.

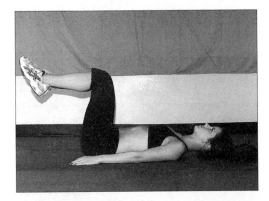

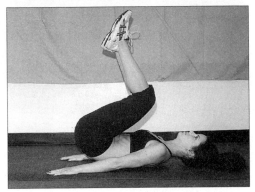

TRAINER'S TIPS

- Make sure your abs are doing the work. Don't rock, using momentum.
- Don't rest your hips on the floor at the end of the movement.
- Keep constant tension on your abs.
- If your hands are at your sides, make sure you're using them just for balance and not to push off.
- Focus your mind on your lower abs.

■ Hip-Ups

DIFFICULTY: 2
LOWER BACK: MODERATE RISK
AREA OF FOCUS: LOWER ABS

STARTING POSITION: Lie flat on your back with your legs extended straight up, perpendicular to your body (knees un-locked). Place your hands at your sides, palms down, and keep your neck long and your head aligned with your spine.

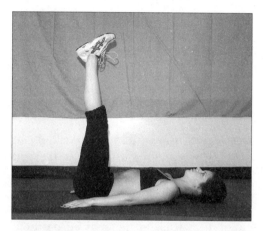

THE MOVE: Use your lower abs to raise your hips off the floor, bringing your hips slightly toward your rib cage. Lower your hips back to the starting position until they lightly touch the floor. Repeat.

TRAINER'S TIPS

- Don't kick up with your legs or push off with your hands to get your hips up—use your ab muscles.
- Hold the contraction at the top of the movement.
- Control both the up and the down phases of the movement.
- Focus your mind on your lower abs.

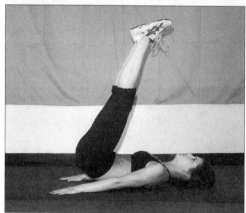

■ Corkscrews

DIFFICULTY: 3
LOWER BACK: HIGH RISK
AREA OF FOCUS: LOWER ABS AND
LOWER OBLIQUES

STARTING POSITION: Lie flat on your back, legs straight and perpendicular to your body (knees unlocked). Place your hands, palms down, at your sides for support.

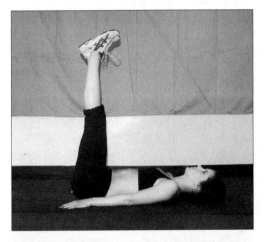

THE MOVE: Raise and twist your hips off the floor in a corkscrew motion to the left. Lower your hips back to the starting position until they lightly touch the floor. Then raise and twist your hips to the right and lower them back to the starting position. Repeat.

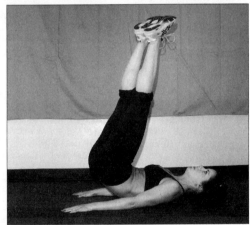

TRAINER'S TIPS

- Don't rest at the bottom of the movement.
- Control both the up and the down phases of the movement.
- Hold the contraction at the top of the movement.
- Don't kick your legs up. Use your abs to elevate them.
- Use your hands for stability, not to push off.
- Focus on your lower abs and obliques.
- Keep your legs perpendicular throughout the exercise. Don't lower them back to the ground.
- Keep your neck lengthened.

■ Knee Raises

DIFFICULTY: 1
LOWER BACK: LOW RISK
AREA OF FOCUS: LOWER ABS

STARTING POSITION: Lie flat on your back, knees bent, both feet on the floor, spine neutral, and neck lengthened.

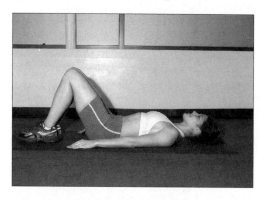

THE MOVE: From this modified position, use your lower abs to draw your knees to your chest. Then lower your legs until your heels lightly touch the floor. Repeat.

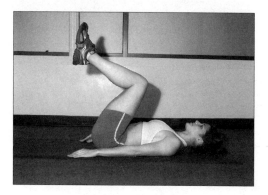

SINGLE-LEG VARIATION: Execute the same movement from the same starting position, but raise only one leg at a time. Complete one side, then switch legs.

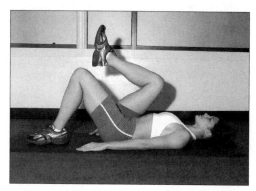

TRAINER'S TIPS

- Concentrate on bringing your knees just to your chest and touching your heels lightly on the floor.
- Don't worry about your hips getting off the floor—they will raise a little naturally when you bring your knees to your chest.
- Hold the contraction at the top of the movement for a count of two.
- Don't let your feet rest at the bottom of the movement.
- This is a good exercise for beginners.

■ Seated Knee Raises

DIFFICULTY: 2
LOWER BACK: LOW RISK
AREA OF FOCUS: LOWER ABS

STARTING POSITION: Sit on the edge of a bench or chair holding on to the back or side of the bench for support, knees bent, heels just off the floor, and upper body upright.

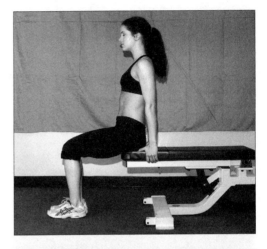

THE MOVE: Use the muscles of your lower abs to draw your knees toward your chest. Then lower in a controlled motion, keeping a bend in your knees. Let your heels lightly brush the floor, then repeat the movement. Keep your upper body stationary during the movement, simply pulling your knees up to your chest. Repeat.

TRAINER'S TIPS

- Control the motion on the way down, keeping tension on your abs.
- Focus your mind on feeling your lower abs do the work.
- Be careful not to lean your torso too far back. Keep it upright.

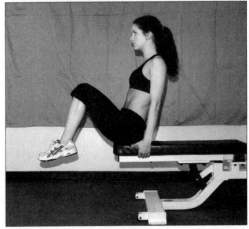

Leg Raises

DIFFICULTY: 2
LOWER BACK: HIGH RISK
AREA OF FOCUS: LOWER ABS

STARTING POSITION: Lie flat on your back, legs extended above your hips, hands at your sides, spine neutral, and neck lengthened.

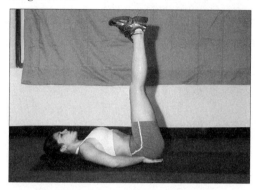

THE MOVE: Use your lower abs to lower your legs toward the floor. Lower your legs only to a distance that will enable you to maintain a neutral spine. This is your range of motion. Then raise your legs in a controlled motion. Repeat.

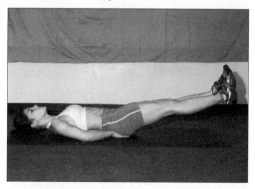

VARIATION ONE: This movement can also be done on an incline board and/or as a single-leg exercise.

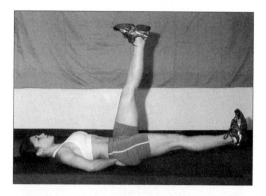

VARIATION TWO: FIGURE EIGHTS: Within your range of motion, draw an imaginary figure eight with your feet. Switch directions after each figure is drawn. Continue until you complete your set.

VARIATION THREE: CRISSCROSSES: Within your range of motion, crisscross your legs back and forth, alternating the top and bottom positions with your legs. Each cross counts as a rep.

TRAINER'S TIPS

- Keep a neutral spine. Don't allow your spine to move out of neutral, creating an exaggerated arch in your lower back.
- Keep your inner core activated.
- Focus your mind on feeling your lower abs do the work.

■ Hanging Knee Raises

DIFFICULTY: 2
LOWER BACK: LOW RISK
AREA OF FOCUS: LOWER ABS

STARTING POSITION: Hang from a bar or vertical chair, legs fully extended.

THE MOVE: Use the muscles of your lower abs to raise your knees to your chest, letting your hips move forward as your knees pass the 90-degree angle. Your feet should hang down below your knees. Then lower them in a controlled motion back to the starting position. Repeat.

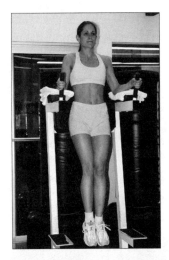

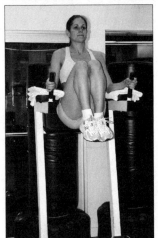

TRAINER'S TIPS

- Bring your knees as high up on your chest as possible.
- When your legs are fully extended at the bottom of the movement, don't rest down there—bring your legs right back up for the next repetition.
- This is a good movement to build strength for Hanging Leg Raises (page 169).
- If you have problems getting your knees up to your chest, don't worry. Your range of motion will improve with work.
- Focus your mind on feeling your lower abs do the work.

■ Hanging Knee Raises: Alternating

DIFFICULTY: 2
LOWER BACK: LOW RISK
AREA OF FOCUS: LOWER ABS

STARTING POSITION: Hang from a bar or vertical chair, legs fully extended.

THE MOVE: Using the muscles of your lower abs, bring your right knee up to your chest, then lower it. Repeat the movement with your left leg. Alternate until you have completed your set.

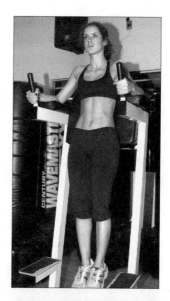

TRAINER'S TIPS

- Bring your knees up as high on your chest as possible.
- Let your hips come forward after your knees pass the 90-degree angle.
- Don't rest at the bottom of the movement—keep constant tension on your abs.
- Focus your mind on feeling your lower abs do the work.
- You may alternate the movement or do multiple repetitions on one side and then switch.

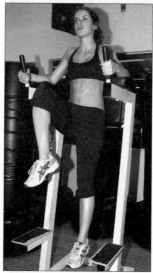

■ Hanging Knee Raises: Bicycles

DIFFICULTY: 2
LOWER BACK: MODERATE RISK
AREA OF FOCUS: LOWER ABS

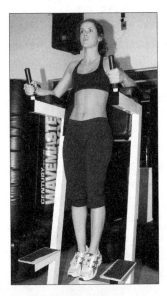

STARTING POSITION: Hang from a bar or vertical chair, legs fully extended.

THE MOVE: Use the muscles of your lower abs to move your legs as if you were pedaling a bicycle. Raise your right knee toward your chest; as you begin to lower it, simultaneously raise your left knee. Your knees should pass each other at the midpoint of the movement. Your left knee continues to your chest, and your right knee completes its downward range of motion. Repeat.

TRAINER'S TIPS

- Bring your knee past your waist.
- Let your hips naturally roll forward when your knee passes through the 90-degree angle.
- Try not to swing too much. Keep the motion controlled.
- Focus your mind on feeling your abs do the work.

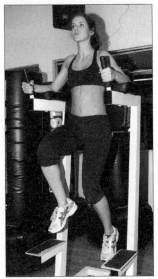

■ Hanging Leg Raises

DIFFICULTY: 3
LOWER BACK: HIGH RISK
AREA OF FOCUS: LOWER ABS

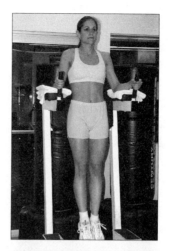

STARTING POSITION: Hang from a bar or vertical chair, legs fully extended.

HALF LEG RAISES: Using the muscles of your lower abs, raise your legs, keeping them straight (knees unlocked) until they are perpendicular with your upper body (at a 90-degree angle). Then lower them in a controlled motion.

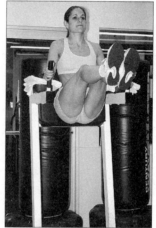

FULL LEG RAISES: Use the muscles of your lower abs to raise your legs (knees unlocked) past the 90-degree angle, curling your hips up toward your rib cage.

SINGLE LEG VARIATION: Use your lower abs to raise one leg at a time.

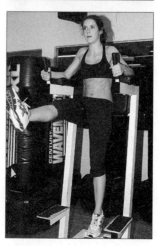

TRAINER'S TIPS

- Lower your legs in a controlled motion. Don't just let them drop.
- Don't use a swinging motion to power your legs up.
- Focus your mind on feeling your lower ab muscles raising and lowering your legs.
- Straight-leg raises activate the hip flexors more than bent-leg raises, but they are good for variety and training the muscle from a new angle.

CHAPTER NINETEEN

Area Two: Obliques

PREVIEW: *This chapter introduces exercises that train your obliques.*

■ ■ ■

■ Crossovers

DIFFICULTY: 2
LOWER BACK: MODERATE RISK
AREA OF FOCUS: OBLIQUES

STARTING POSITION: Lie flat on your back, knees bent and both feet on the floor. Then cross your right ankle over your left knee, making a triangle between your legs. Your left hand goes behind your head, elbow extended. Your right hand can either rest extended at your right side or, preferably, rest on your left side, so you can feel your obliques work.

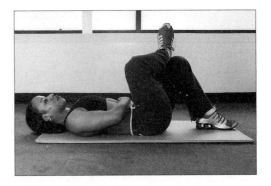

THE MOVE: Use your abs to raise and cross your left shoulder toward your right knee. Lower your body back to the starting position until your shoulder blades lightly touch the floor. Repeat the movement to the other side.

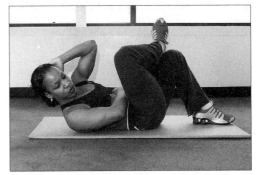

TRAINER'S TIPS

- Make sure your torso twists toward your knee. Don't just reach with your elbow.
- Make sure you are also raising your torso up, not just rolling to the side.
- Control both the up and the down phases of the movement.
- Hold the contraction at the top of the movement.
- Focus your mind on your obliques.

■ Catches

DIFFICULTY: 1
LOWER BACK: LOW RISK
AREA OF FOCUS: OBLIQUES

STARTING POSITION: Lie flat on your back, knees bent, both feet on the floor, and your arms extended toward your knees.

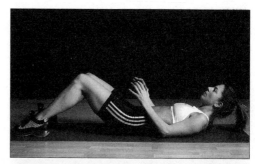

THE MOVE: Use your ab muscles to raise your torso diagonally, bringing your right shoulder across the centerline of your body and both hands outside and above your left knee, as if you were going to catch a ball. Lower your torso back to the starting position. Repeat the movement to your right side.

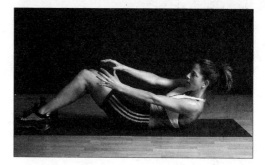

TRAINER'S TIPS

- Make sure you get both arms outside your knee and slightly above knee level.
- Keep your lower back supported on the floor.
- Focus your mind on your oblique muscles as you cross from side to side.

■ Double Side Leg Raises

DIFFICULTY: 3
LOWER BACK: LOW RISK
AREA OF FOCUS: OBLIQUES

STARTING POSITION: Lie on your side, resting on your hip, both legs extended straight. Rest on your tricep for support.

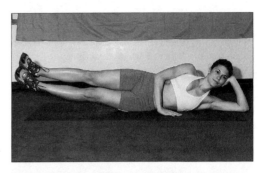

THE MOVE: Using your oblique muscles, raise both legs off the floor as high as you can lift them. Then lower them back down, lightly touching the floor. Repeat the movement until you have completed your set. Then switch sides.

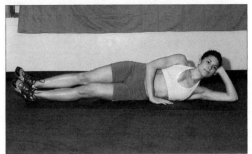

TRAINER'S TIPS

- Concentrate on using just your abs. Don't recruit other muscles to help you out.
- Control your legs on the way down.
- Don't rest your legs on the floor at the bottom of the movement. Keep constant tension on your abs.

■ Side Jackknives

DIFFICULTY: 2
LOWER BACK: LOW RISK
AREA OF FOCUS: OBLIQUES

STARTING POSITION: Lie on your left hip, legs together. Place your right hand behind your right ear and your left hand on your right side.

THE MOVE: Use your oblique muscles to simultaneously raise your top leg and your torso, bringing them together. Repeat the movement until you have completed your set. Then reverse the procedure for the opposite side.

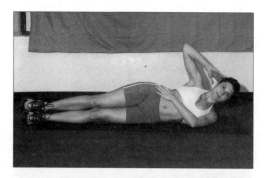

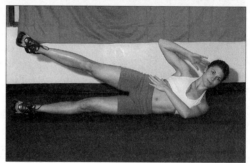

TRAINER'S TIPS

- Bring your leg slightly forward to increase your range of motion.
- Focus your mind on feeling your obliques do the work.
- Make sure your upper body moves off the floor. Don't move just your head.
- Don't rest your leg and torso at the bottom of the movement.

■ Double Side Jackknives

DIFFICULTY: 3
LOWER BACK: MODERATE RISK
AREA OF FOCUS: OBLIQUES

STARTING POSITION: Lie on your right hip, legs together and fully extended. Place your right elbow against your body for support and your left hand behind your left ear.

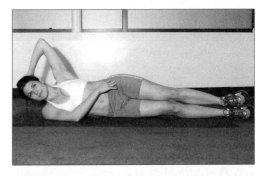

THE MOVE: Use your oblique muscles to raise both legs and simultaneously bring your torso up. Lower your body in a controlled motion and repeat. Then reverse the procedure for the opposite side.

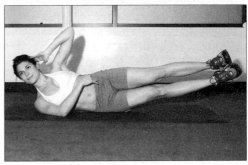

TRAINER'S TIPS

- Bring your legs slightly forward to increase your range of motion.
- Focus your mind on feeling your obliques do the work.
- Make sure your upper body moves off the floor. Don't move just your head.

■ Side Sit-Ups: Roman Chair

DIFFICULTY: 3
LOWER BACK: MODERATE RISK
AREA OF FOCUS: OBLIQUES

STARTING POSITION: Secure yourself in a Roman chair, resting your left hip against the support. Then straighten your body and place your hands behind your head.

THE MOVE: Lower your torso, keeping your body turned to the side. Then, using your obliques, raise your torso back to the starting position. Repeat. Then execute the movement on the opposite side.

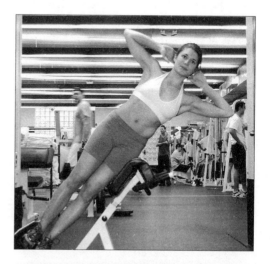

TRAINER'S TIPS

- To increase the intensity of the movement, bring your hands behind your head.
- Control the motion on the way down. Don't just let yourself drop.
- Don't rest at the top of the movement.
- Focus your mind on feeling your abs and obliques do the work.

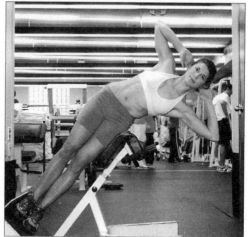

■ Side Bends with Weight

DIFFICULTY: 1
LOWER BACK: MODERATE RISK
AREA OF FOCUS: OBLIQUES

STARTING POSITION: Stand upright, feet shoulder-width apart, knees unlocked, and hands at your sides holding dumbbells.

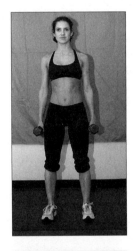

THE MOVE: Bend to the side and lower the left dumbbell down your right leg (resisting your oblique muscles) until you feel a good stretch. Then, using your obliques, raise the weight back to the starting position. Alternate sides.

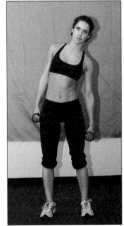

TRAINER'S TIPS

- Concentrate on feeling your obliques raise and lower the weight.
- Using heavy weights will build muscle mass. So you will probably want to use light weights and do this exercise only periodically.
- Don't rest at the top of the movement.

■ Standing Twists

DIFFICULTY: 1
LOWER BACK: LOW RISK
AREA OF FOCUS: OBLIQUES

STARTING POSITION: Stand upright, feet a little wider than shoulder width, and place your hands behind your ears.

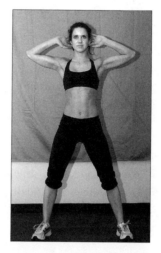

THE MOVE: Keeping your hips stationary, use your oblique muscles to twist your torso to the left as far as it can go; then twist back to the right through a full range of motion. Repeat.

TRAINER'S TIPS

- Keep a slow, controlled motion at the beginning of your set. Then, as you get looser, you can pick up the pace.
- Don't turn your hips. Keep them stable. Your range of motion will be determined by how far you can twist without letting your hips start to turn.
- If you have lower-back problems, you should keep the motion slow and controlled.
- Keep in constant motion during this movement.

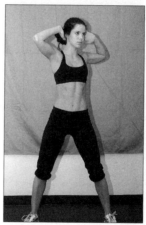

■ Bent-Knee Leg-Overs: Single Leg

DIFFICULTY: 1
LOWER BACK: LOW RISK
AREA OF FOCUS: OBLIQUES

STARTING POSITION: Lie flat on your back, hands spread out perpendicular to your body, left leg fully extended, and right leg bent at a 90-degree angle to your body, with your lower leg extended out.

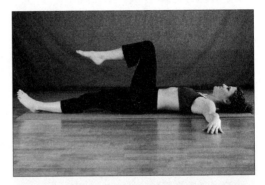

THE MOVE: Use your oblique muscles to cross your right knee over your body, lightly touching the floor on the opposite side. Then cross it back over to the starting position. Repeat the movement until you have completed your set. Then switch legs.

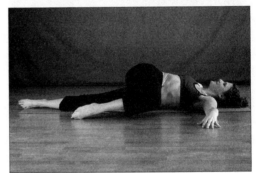

TRAINER'S TIPS

- As you cross your leg over, allow your hip to roll with the motion.
- Concentrate on feeling your obliques do the work.
- Make sure you keep the lower half of your leg extended out during the movement.
- Keep both shoulder blades on the floor throughout the movement.
- Think of having your leg, hip, and obliques fused together, so they move as a single unit.

■ Leg-Overs: Single Leg

DIFFICULTY: 2
LOWER BACK: MODERATE RISK
AREA OF FOCUS: OBLIQUES

STARTING POSITION: Lie flat on your back, hands spread out perpendicular to your body, left leg fully extended, and right leg straight up.

THE MOVE: Use your oblique muscles to cross your right leg toward your left hand. Lightly touch the floor with your foot; then cross the leg back to the straight-up starting position. Repeat the movement until you have completed your set. Then switch legs.

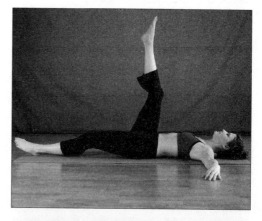

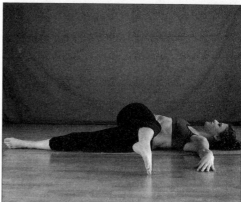

TRAINER'S TIPS

- As you cross your leg over, allow your hip to roll with the motion.
- Concentrate on feeling your abs do the work.
- If you can't move your leg to the straight-up position, choose a position that is comfortable. Your flexibility will improve.
- Think of having your leg, hip, and obliques fused together, so they move as a single unit.
- Keep both shoulder blades on the floor throughout the movement.

■ Bent-Knee Leg-Overs: Double Leg

DIFFICULTY: 2
LOWER BACK: LOW RISK
AREA OF FOCUS: OBLIQUES

STARTING POSITION: Lie flat on your back, hands spread out perpendicular to your body. Raise your knees directly above your hips, lower legs extended parallel to the floor.

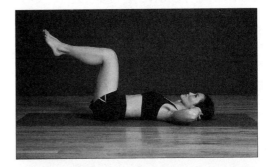

THE MOVE: Use your oblique muscles to lower both knees to your left side, so the outside of your left thigh gently touches the floor, then raise your knees back to the starting position. Repeat the movement to the opposite side.

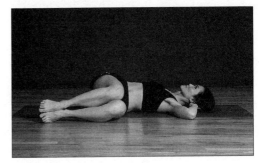

TRAINER'S TIPS

- As you lower your legs to the side, let your hips roll in the same direction.
- Keep both shoulder blades on the floor throughout the movement.
- Focus on feeling your obliques do the work.
- Keep your neck lengthened.

■ Leg-Overs: Double Leg

DIFFICULTY: 3
LOWER BACK: MODERATE RISK
AREA OF FOCUS: OBLIQUES

STARTING POSITION: Lie flat on your back, hands spread out perpendicular to your body and both legs extended straight up.

THE MOVE: Use your oblique muscles to lower both legs to your left side until your feet lightly touch the floor, then raise your legs back to the starting position. Repeat the movement to the opposite side.

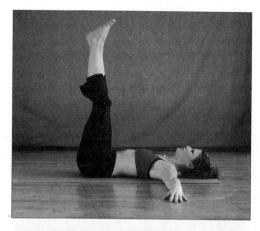

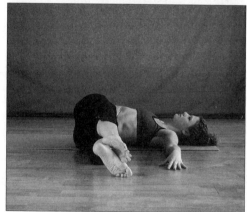

TRAINER'S TIPS

- As you lower both legs to the side, let your hips roll in that direction with the motion.
- Try to lower your legs at a 90-degree angle from your upper body.
- If you can't move your legs to the straight-up position or lower them at a 90-degree angle, take them to an angle that is comfortable. Your flexibility will improve.
- Keep your shoulders and back flat on the floor throughout the entire movement.
- Concentrate on feeling your ab muscles do the work.
- This movement is the most difficult of the leg-over series, so work up to it, gradually building strength with the other movements first.

■ Lying Side Bends

DIFFICULTY: 1
LOWER BACK: LOW RISK
AREA OF FOCUS: OBLIQUES

STARTING POSITION: Lie flat on your back, knees bent, both feet on the floor, hands behind your ears.

THE MOVE: Use your oblique muscles to bend your elbow to your hip. Then straighten your torso back to the starting position. Repeat to the same side or alternate.

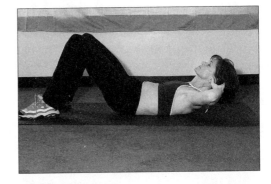

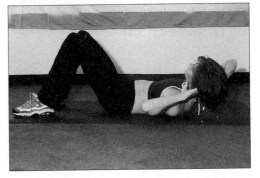

TRAINER'S TIPS

- Focus your mind on feeling your obliques bend your body.
- Hold the contraction at the top of the movement for a count of two.
- Keep your elbow close to the floor as you make a semicircle toward your hip.

■ Heel Touches

DIFFICULTY: 1
LOWER BACK: LOW RISK
AREA OF FOCUS: OBLIQUES

STARTING POSITION: Lie flat on your back, knees bent, both feet on the floor, and hands at your sides.

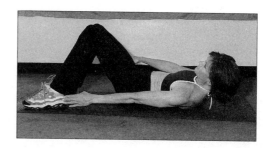

THE MOVE: As you raise your shoulder blades about an inch off the floor, bend to the left, touching your left heel with your left hand. Then bend the other way, touching your right heel with your right hand.

TRAINER'S TIPS

- Focus your mind on feeling your obliques bend your body.
- Feel your body bend at your waist as you touch your heel.
- Keep your shoulder blades off the floor for the entire movement.

CHAPTER TWENTY

Area Three: Upper Abs

PREVIEW: *This chapter introduces exercises to train your upper abs.*

■ ■ ■

■ Crunches: Knees Bent

DIFFICULTY: 1
LOWER BACK: LOW RISK
AREA OF FOCUS: UPPER ABS

STARTING POSITION: Lie flat on your back, knees bent, both feet on the floor, and hands in the position of choice.

THE MOVE: Use your upper abs to raise your shoulder blades off the floor in a forward curling motion. Then lower your shoulders to the starting position, lightly touching your shoulder blades to the floor. Repeat.

VARIATION: You can also do the crunch movement on an incline board.

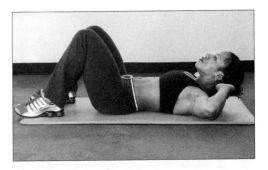

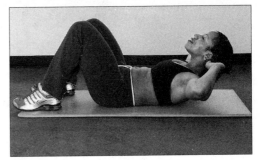

TRAINER'S TIPS

- Keep constant tension on your abs throughout the movement.
- Focus your mind on feeling your upper abs do the work.
- Don't rest at the bottom of the movement.
- Make sure you move your shoulder blades off the floor. Don't move just your neck and head.
- Keep a neutral spine.

■ Crunches: Knees Up

DIFFICULTY: 1
LOWER BACK: LOW RISK
AREA OF FOCUS: UPPER ABS

STARTING POSITION: Lie flat on your back and raise your legs so your thighs are perpendicular to your body, placing your calves and feet parallel to the floor and your hands in the position of choice.

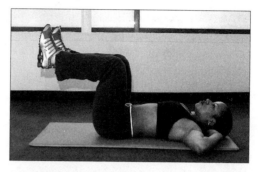

THE MOVE: Use the muscles of your upper abs to raise your shoulder blades and back off the floor in a forward curling motion. Then lower your torso to the starting position, lightly touching your shoulder blades to the floor. Repeat.

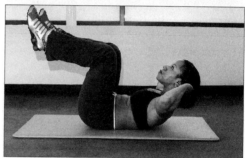

TRAINER'S TIPS

- Get your shoulder blades off the floor with each repetition. Don't move just your neck and head.
- Keep the movement controlled.
- Don't rest your shoulders on the floor at the bottom of the movement.
- Focus your mind on feeling your upper abs do the work.
- Keep a neutral spine.

■ Butterfly Crunches

DIFFICULTY: 1
LOWER BACK: LOW RISK
AREA OF FOCUS: UPPER ABS

STARTING POSITION: Lying flat on your back, bring the soles of your feet together and let your knees fall to the sides. Place your hands in the position of choice.

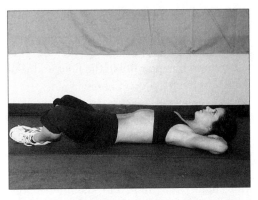

THE MOVE: Raise your shoulder blades off the floor two to three inches by curling your rib cage toward your hips. Hold the contraction at the top of the movement. Then lower your shoulder blades back to the starting position. Repeat the movement.

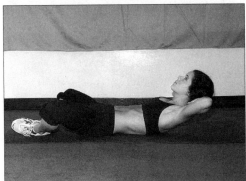

TRAINER'S TIPS

- Keep constant tension on your abs.
- Focus your mind on feeling your upper abs do the work.
- Don't rest at the bottom of the movement.
- Make sure you move your shoulder blades off the floor. Don't move just your neck and head.
- Keep a neutral spine.
- As in other crunch variations, this leg position adds variety and hits the muscle from a different angle, shocking the muscle and giving it better overall development.

■ Toe Touches

DIFFICULTY: 1
LOWER BACK: LOW RISK
AREA OF FOCUS: UPPER ABS

STARTING POSITION: Lie flat on your back, legs straight up and perpendicular to your body (knees unlocked) and arms extended straight up.

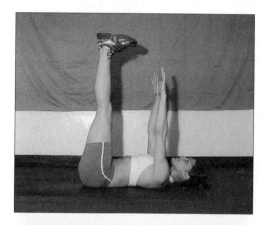

THE MOVE: Use your upper abs to raise your hands toward your toes. Then lower your torso back to the starting position, letting your shoulder blades lightly touch the floor. Repeat.

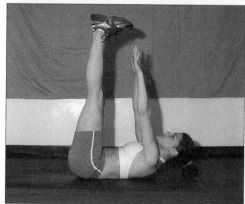

TRAINER'S TIPS

- Don't rest at the bottom of the movement. When you feel your shoulder blades touch the floor, start the next repetition.
- Don't worry about actually touching your toes. The objective is to get your shoulder blades off the floor two or three inches.
- If you have problems holding your legs perpendicular, get them as close as you can or hold them up against a wall.
- Keep your neck lengthened.

■ Crunches:
Legs Straight Out

DIFFICULTY: 2
LOWER BACK: MODERATE RISK
AREA OF FOCUS: UPPER ABS

STARTING POSITION: Lie flat on your back, legs extended straight out on the floor (knees unlocked) and hands in the position of choice.

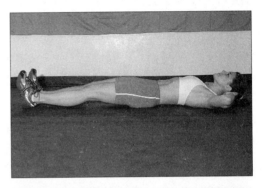

THE MOVE: Use the muscles of your upper abs to raise your shoulder blades off the floor in a forward curling motion. Then lower your shoulder blades to the starting position, lightly touching the floor. Repeat.

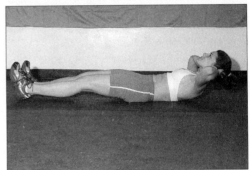

TRAINER'S TIPS

- Make sure you keep your knees unlocked so your thigh muscles aren't contracting.
- Turn your knees slightly out.
- Keep constant tension on your abs throughout the movement.
- Don't rest at the bottom of the movement.
- Focus your mind on feeling your upper abs do the work.
- Make sure you move your shoulder blades off the floor. Don't move just your neck and head.
- Keep a neutral spine.

■ Crunches: Raised Hips

DIFFICULTY: 2
LOWER BACK: MODERATE RISK
AREA OF FOCUS: UPPER ABS

STARTING POSITION: Lie flat on your back, knees bent and feet flat on the floor. Place your hands in the position of choice, pushing your hips up toward the ceiling (about six inches off the floor), so your buttocks are contracted. Hold this position throughout the exercise.

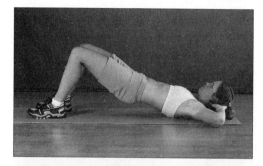

THE MOVE: Use your upper abs to raise your shoulder blades off the floor. Lower and repeat. You will probably get only one to three inches of movement, so don't be discouraged.

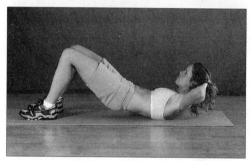

TRAINER'S TIPS

- Keep constant tension on your abs throughout the movement.
- Focus your mind on feeling your upper abs do the work.
- Don't rest at the bottom of the movement.
- Make sure you move your shoulder blades off the floor. Don't move just your neck and head.
- Keep the movement controlled.

■ Crunches: Split Leg

DIFFICULTY: 1
LOWER BACK: MODERATE RISK
AREA OF FOCUS: UPPER ABS AND
   OBLIQUES

STARTING POSITION: Lie flat on your back, left leg straight up and perpendicular to your body (knee unlocked), right leg extended on the floor (knee unlocked), and hands in the position of choice.

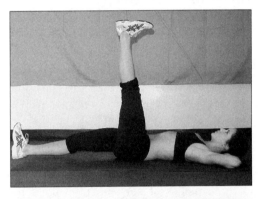

THE MOVE: Use your ab muscles to raise your chest toward your left knee in a curling motion. Then lower yourself until your shoulder blades lightly touch the floor. Repeat. Alternate legs with each repetition.

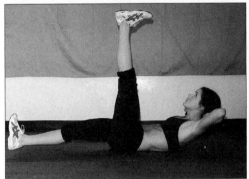

TRAINER'S TIPS

- Get your shoulder blades off the floor with each repetition. Don't move just your neck and head.
- Don't rest at the bottom of the movement. When your shoulder blades touch the floor, start the next repetition.
- Focus your mind on feeling your abs do the work.
- Keep a neutral spine. Do not rock.

■ Crunches:
Legs Straight Out, V-Spread

DIFFICULTY: 2
LOWER BACK: MODERATE RISK
AREA OF FOCUS: UPPER ABS

STARTING POSITION: Lie flat on your back, legs extended straight out on the floor (knees unlocked) and hands in the position of choice. Spread your legs wide.

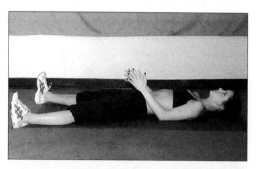

THE MOVE: Use the muscles of your upper abs to raise your shoulder blades off the floor in a forward curling motion over your left leg. Then lower your shoulder blades to the starting position, lightly touching the floor. Repeat.

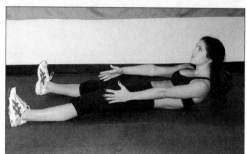

TRAINER'S TIPS

- Make sure to keep your knees unlocked so your thigh muscles aren't contracting.
- Turn your knees slightly out.
- Keep constant tension on your abs throughout the movement.
- Don't rest at the bottom of the movement.
- Focus your mind on feeling your upper abs do the work.
- Make sure you move your shoulder blades off the floor. Don't move just your neck and head.

■ Bench Crunches

DIFFICULTY: 2
LOWER BACK: MODERATE RISK
AREA OF FOCUS: UPPER ABS

STARTING POSITION: Lie on your back on a bench, bending your knees, placing both feet flat on the bench. Then position your shoulder blades so they drop over the edge of the bench, and support your head with the hand position of choice.

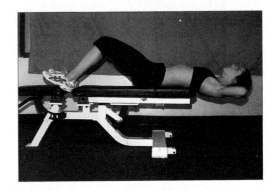

THE MOVE: Use your upper abs to raise and curl your torso up and over the bench toward your rib cage. Then lower your shoulder blades below the bench and repeat.

TRAINER'S TIPS

- Keep constant tension on your abs throughout the full range of motion (both raising and lowering).
- Make sure you lower your shoulder blades below the bench on each repetition.
- Raise your torso as high as you would on a normal crunch.
- Don't rest at the bottom of the movement.
- Focus your mind on your upper abs.

■ Cable Crunches

DIFFICULTY: 3
LOWER BACK: LOW RISK
AREA OF FOCUS: UPPER ABS

STARTING POSITION: Grab the cable pull-down attachment, then kneel facing the cable machine, hips up, holding the attachment to your forehead with both hands.

THE MOVE: Use your upper abs to bend forward. Bring your head down and out over you knees, driving your elbows to your knees while keeping the cable tight and held stationary at your forehead. Come up to approximately a 45-degree angle. Repeat.

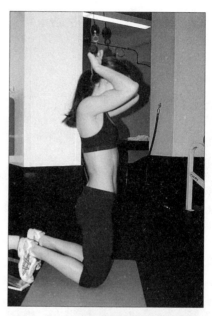

TRAINER'S TIPS

- Raise and lower the weights in a controlled motion. Don't pop back up.
- Don't come all the way up on each repetition—maintain approximately the 45-degree angle. Hold the contraction at the bottom of the movement.
- Imagine that you are bending over a bar that is the height of your upper abs.

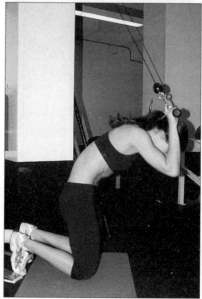

■ Crunches: Figure 4

DIFFICULTY: 2
LOWER BACK: LOW RISK
AREA OF FOCUS: UPPER ABS

STARTING POSITION: Lie flat on your back, place your left ankle across your right knee, then raise your right leg off the ground, bringing your knee over your hip.

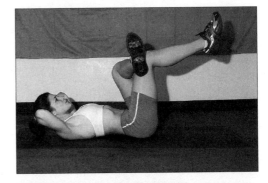

THE MOVE: Use the muscles of your upper abs to raise your shoulder blades off the floor in a forward curling motion. Then lower your torso to the starting position, lightly touching your shoulder blades to the floor. Repeat the movement until you have completed your set. Then switch legs.

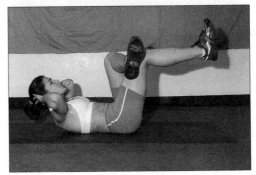

TRAINER'S TIPS

- Keep constant tension on your abs throughout the movement.
- Focus your mind on feeling your upper abs do the work.
- Don't rest at the bottom of the movement.
- Make sure you move your shoulder blades off the floor. Don't move just your neck and head.

■ Knee Touches

DIFFICULTY: 1
LOWER BACK: LOW RISK
AREA OF FOCUS: UPPER ABS

STARTING POSITION: Lie flat on your back, knees bent, both feet on the floor, and hands pointing up.

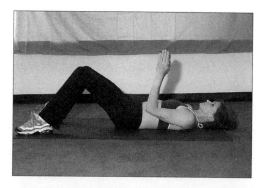

THE MOVE: Use the muscles of your upper abs to raise your shoulder blades off the floor as you bring your hands forward to touch the tops of your knees. Repeat.

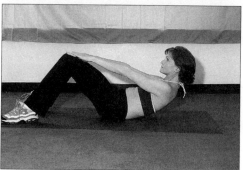

TRAINER'S TIPS

- Keep constant tension on your abs throughout the movement.
- Focus your mind on feeling your upper abs do the work.
- Don't rest at the bottom of the movement.
- Make sure you move your shoulder blades off the floor. Don't move just your neck and head.

■ Crunches on Side

DIFFICULTY: 1
LOWER BACK: LOW RISK
AREA OF FOCUS: UPPER ABS

STARTING POSITION: Lie on your side in a fetal position, one knee on top of the other.

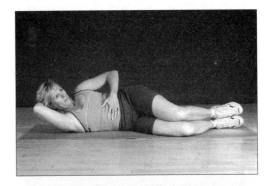

THE MOVE: Curl your rib cage toward your hips. Repeat the movement until you have completed your set. Then switch sides.

TRAINER'S TIPS

- Keep constant tension on your abs throughout the movement.
- Focus your mind on feeling your upper abs do the work.
- Hold the contraction at the top of the movement for a count of two.
- Keep your neck lengthened.

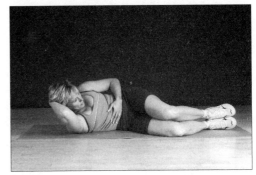

CHAPTER TWENTY-ONE

Area Four: Combination Exercises

PREVIEW: *This chapter introduces exercises that emphasize more than one area.*

■ ■ ■

■ Bicycles

DIFFICULTY: 2
LOWER BACK: MODERATE RISK
AREA OF FOCUS: UPPER AND LOWER
    ABS AND OBLIQUES

STARTING POSITION: Lie flat on your back, knees bent and your feet on the floor, and hands behind your ears.

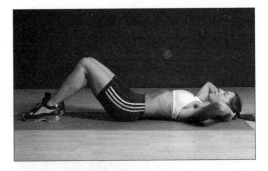

THE MOVE: Use your abs to simultaneously bring your right shoulder and your left knee toward each other. Then extend your left leg as you cross your right shoulder to your left knee. Repeat in a fluid motion to the opposite side. Keep the motion continuous, as if you were pedaling a bicycle.

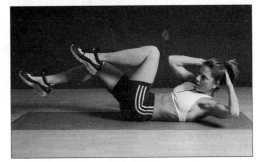

TRAINER'S TIPS

- Keep the motion controlled. Don't go too fast.
- Make sure your entire torso twists. Don't move just your elbow to your knee.
- Make sure your shoulder blades come off the floor each time.
- Don't let your legs touch the floor.
- Focus your mind on feeling your abs do the work.
- Keep the small of your back pressed against the floor and maintain a stable position. Do not rock.

■ Crunch Circles

DIFFICULTY: 2
LOWER BACK: MODERATE RISK
AREA OF FOCUS:
UPPER ABS AND OBLIQUES

STARTING POSITION: Lie flat on your back, knees bent, both feet on the floor, and hands in the position of choice.

THE MOVE: Use your upper abs to curl your torso toward your rib cage in a small circular motion. If your torso were a hand on a clock, starting position would be six o'clock; moving up and around to twelve o'clock (position of a normal crunch) and back down and around to six o'clock completes one repetition. Alternate directions with each repetition.

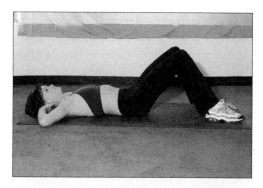

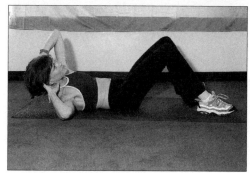

TRAINER'S TIPS

- Keep constant tension on your abs throughout the full range of motion (all directions).
- Raise your torso as high as you would for a normal crunch.
- Don't rest at the bottom of the movement.
- Focus your mind on your abs.

■ Reverse Crunch Circles

DIFFICULTY: 3
LOWER BACK: MODERATE RISK
AREA OF FOCUS:
   LOWER ABS AND OBLIQUES

STARTING POSITION: Lie flat on your back, positioning your legs so your thighs are perpendicular to your body and your lower legs are parallel to the floor.

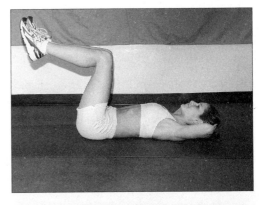

THE MOVE: Use your lower abs to curl your hips toward your rib cage in a small circular motion. If your hips were a hand on a clock, starting position would be six o'clock; moving up and around to twelve o'clock (position of a normal reverse crunch) and back down and around to six o'clock completes one repetition. Alternate directions with each repetition.

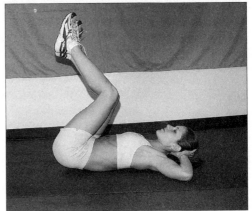

TRAINER'S TIPS

- Keep constant tension on your abs throughout the full range of motion (all directions).
- Raise your hips as high as you would for a normal reverse crunch.
- Don't rest at the bottom of the movement.
- Focus your mind on your abs.

■ Double Crunches

DIFFICULTY: 2
LOWER BACK: MODERATE RISK
AREA OF FOCUS:
  LOWER AND UPPER ABS

STARTING POSITION: Lie flat on your back, knees bent, both feet on the floor, and hands behind your ears.

THE MOVE: Use your abs to simultaneously raise your torso and your legs toward each other. Lower your back to the starting position. Repeat.

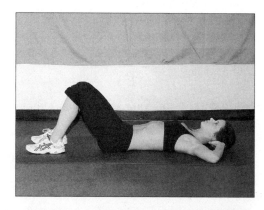

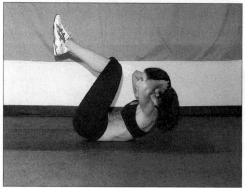

TRAINER'S TIPS

- Concentrate on keeping constant tension on your abs.
- Focus your mind on feeling your abs do the work.
- Don't let your shoulder blades or feet rest on the floor at the completion of each repetition.
- Let your heels lightly touch the floor on each rep.

■ Double Crunches with a Cross

DIFFICULTY: 3
LOWER BACK: HIGH RISK
AREA OF FOCUS: UPPER AND LOWER ABS AND OBLIQUES

STARTING POSITION: Lie flat on your back with your knees bent and your feet flat on the floor.

THE MOVE: Using your ab muscles, simultaneously bring both knees toward your left shoulder while curling the shoulder toward your knees. Lower your body back to the starting position. Repeat the movement to the opposite side.

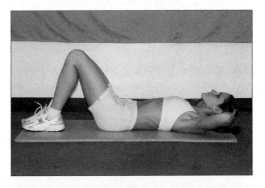

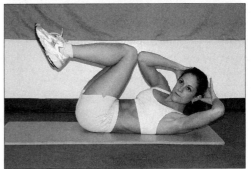

TRAINER'S TIPS

- Concentrate on keeping constant tension on your abs.
- Focus your mind on feeling your abs do the work.
- Don't let your leg touch the floor at the bottom of the movement.
- When returning to the starting position, maintain a straight back—do not arch.

■ Crunches with a Twist

DIFFICULTY: 2
LOWER BACK: MODERATE RISK
AREA OF FOCUS:
  UPPER ABS AND OBLIQUES

STARTING POSITION: Lie flat on your back, knees bent, both feet on the floor, and hands in the position of choice.

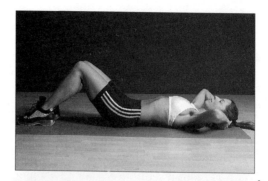

THE MOVE: Use your upper ab muscles to twist your right shoulder toward your left knee in a forward curling motion, so your shoulder blades come off the floor. Repeat the movement to the opposite side.

VARIATIONS: You can incorporate this twisting movement (activating the oblique muscles) into all the crunch variations: butterfly crunches; knees up; legs straight out; legs straight up; raised hips; and on an incline board.

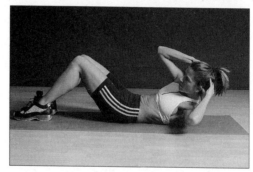

TRAINER'S TIPS

• Keep constant tension on your abs. Don't rest at the bottom of the movement.
• Keep the movement isolated to your upper abs and your obliques. Don't come up too high.
• Focus your mind on feeling your abs do the work.
• Keep a neutral spine.
• The top range of motion is complete when the nonworking shoulder blade comes slightly off the floor.
• On an incline board, increase the slant as your strength increases.

■ Oblique Crunches

DIFFICULTY: 2
LOWER BACK: MODERATE RISK
AREA OF FOCUS: UPPER AND LOWER
  ABS AND OBLIQUES

STARTING POSITION: Lie flat on your back, letting both your legs fall to the left side so you're resting on your right hip. If your top leg won't go all the way down, let it rest in a comfortable position as close to the other leg as possible.

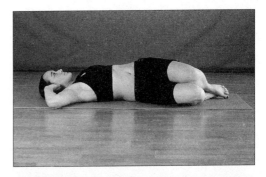

THE MOVE: Keeping your shoulders as close to parallel to the floor as possible, use your ab muscles to raise both shoulder blades off the floor, bringing your rib cage toward your pelvis. Then lower your torso in a controlled motion. Repeat the movement with your legs on the opposite side.

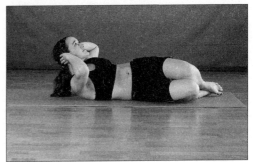

TRAINER'S TIPS

- Focus your mind on feeling your abs do the work.
- Keep constant tension on your abs.
- Don't rest at the bottom of the movement.
- Make sure you move your shoulder blades off the floor. Don't move just your neck and head.
- Try not to lead the movement with a single shoulder. Keep your shoulders parallel to the floor.

■ Toe Touches with a Twist

DIFFICULTY: 2
LOWER BACK: MODERATE RISK
**AREA OF FOCUS: UPPER AND LOWER
  ABS AND OBLIQUES**

STARTING POSITION: Lie flat on your back, legs straight up (knees unlocked) and perpendicular to your body, arms extended toward the ceiling.

THE MOVE: Use your abs to raise your right shoulder off the floor, touching the outside of your left little toe with your right hand. Lower your shoulder back to the floor and repeat the movement to the opposite side, touching your left hand to the outside of your right little toe.

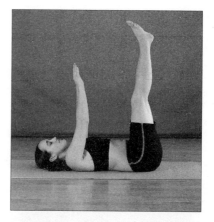

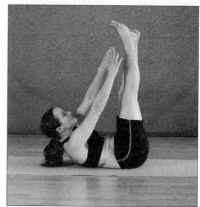

TRAINER'S TIPS

• Concentrate on feeling your abs do the work.
• Keep the movement controlled. Don't jerk up to reach your toes.
• Don't rest at the bottom of the movement. Keep tension on your abs.
• If you can't touch your toes, just reach as far as you can. Your range of motion will improve with work.
• Keep a neutral spine.

■ Russian Twists

DIFFICULTY: 3
LOWER BACK: HIGH RISK
AREA OF FOCUS: UPPER AND LOWER
   ABS AND OBLIQUES

STARTING POSITION: Find a position of balance on your buttocks, feet in the air extended halfway out and hands clasped and extended out in front of you.

THE MOVE: From this position, twist side to side while maintaining your balance on your buttocks, keeping constant tension on your abs. Repeat.

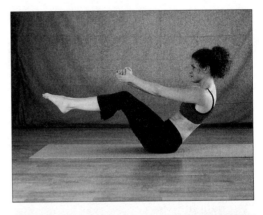

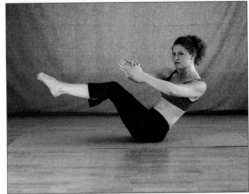

TRAINER'S TIPS

- Don't crunch your body together. Keep good posture and try to relax into the position.
- Go through a full range of motion, twisting as far to your right as you can, then as far to your left as you can.
- Your neck and head should remain lengthened and aligned with the rest of your spine.
- Don't move your head from side to side.
- Maintain a stable position on your buttocks.

■ Russian Twists: Roman Chair

DIFFICULTY: 2
LOWER BACK: HIGH RISK
**AREA OF FOCUS: UPPER AND LOWER
ABS AND OBLIQUES**

STARTING POSITION: Sit on a Roman chair, put your feet under the support handles, and lean back to approximately a 45-degree angle, so you feel tension on you upper and lower abs. Extend your hands out in front of you and clasp them together. You can also do this exercise holding a broom handle or a light pole across the back of your shoulders.

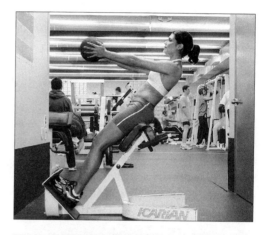

THE MOVE: From this position, twist to your right, then back to your left, while keeping constant tension on your abs. Repeat.

TRAINER'S TIPS

- Don't crunch your body together—lengthen it and relax.
- Go through a full range of motion, twisting as far to your right as you can, then as far to your left as you can.

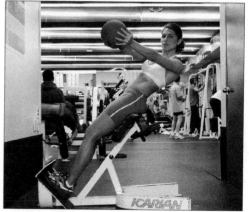

■ Oblique Crosses: V-Spread (Legs Up)

DIFFICULTY: 2
LOWER BACK: HIGH RISK
**AREA OF FOCUS: UPPER AND LOWER
  ABS AND OBLIQUES**

STARTING POSITION: Lie flat on your back, legs fully extended on the floor and spread in a V position (knees unlocked) and hands in the position of choice.

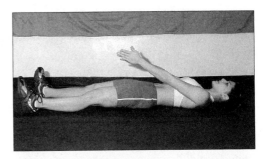

THE MOVE: Lift your left leg off the floor about twelve inches. Then use your ab muscles to raise your torso over your raised leg. Lower your torso and leg to the starting position. Repeat the movement until you have completed your set. Then switch legs.

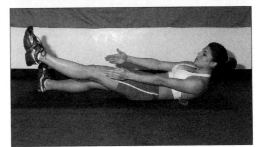

TRAINER'S TIPS

- Make sure you cross your torso toward the leg, contracting the obliques.
- Keep constant tension on your abs.
- Don't rest on the floor after lowering your shoulders.
- Focus your mind on feeling your abs do the work.
- Keep a neutral spine.

▪ V-Ups

DIFFICULTY: 3
LOWER BACK: HIGH RISK
AREA OF FOCUS:
   UPPER AND LOWER ABS

STARTING POSITION: Lie flat on your back, legs fully extended (knees unlocked), heels resting on the floor, and arms extended over your head.

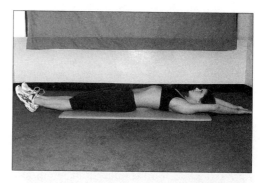

THE MOVE: Use your abs to simultaneously raise your torso and legs together. Then, in a controlled motion, lower your legs and torso back to the starting position. Repeat.

BENT-KNEE VARIATION: Same starting position, except you have your knees bent and your feet flat on the floor. The movement is the same, except you keep your knees bent throughout the range of motion and you end each repetition in a bent-knee position.

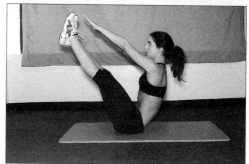

TRAINER'S TIPS

- Focus on feeling your abs pull your torso and legs together.
- Keep the movement controlled— don't jerk yourself up.
- Don't rest your arms and legs at the bottom of the movement.
- Focus your mind on feeling your abs do the work.
- The bent-knee version is easier and puts less stress on your back.

■ V-Ups with a Cross

DIFFICULTY: 3
LOWER BACK: HIGH RISK
AREA OF FOCUS: UPPER AND LOWER
  ABS AND OBLIQUES

STARTING POSITION: Lie flat on your back, legs fully extended (knees unlocked), heels resting on the floor, and arms extended over your head.

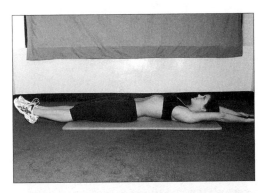

THE MOVE: Use your abs to simultaneously bring your feet and hands together. As you raise your torso and legs, cross your right shoulder toward your left knee and your left knee toward your right shoulder. Then simultaneously lower your legs and torso. Repeat.

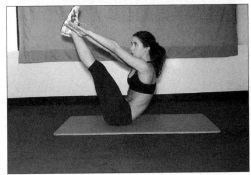

TRAINER'S TIPS

- Think of raising your legs a split second before your torso.
- Keep constant tension on your abs throughout the full range of motion (all directions).
- Don't rest at the bottom of the movement.
- Keep your legs straight (but don't lock your knees).
- Focus your mind on your abs.
- On each side, bring your hands outside your feet.

■ Side Double Crunches

DIFFICULTY: 2
LOWER BACK: MODERATE RISK
**AREA OF FOCUS: UPPER AND LOWER
  ABS AND OBLIQUES**

STARTING POSITION: Lie on your right buttock, legs fully extended (knees unlocked), right arm out front for support, and left hand behind your left ear.

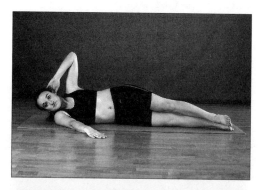

THE MOVE: Use your abs to simultaneously raise your legs and torso off the floor, bringing your knees and chest together. Then return to the starting position. Repeat the movement until you have completed your set. Then switch sides.

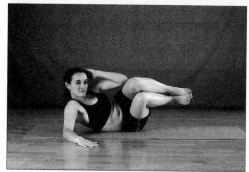

TRAINER'S TIPS

- Don't let your legs and torso rest on the floor at the bottom of the movement.
- Focus your mind on feeling your abs do the work.
- Don't pull your head forward with your hand.

■ Hanging Leg Raises with a Cross: Both Legs

DIFFICULTY: 2
LOWER BACK: MODERATE RISK
AREA OF FOCUS: UPPER AND LOWER ABS AND OBLIQUES

STARTING POSITION: Hang from straps or a vertical chair with your legs fully extended.

THE MOVE: Use your abs to raise and cross both legs (knees unlocked) to the outside of your left hand. Then lower your legs back to the starting position. Repeat the movement to the opposite side, bringing your legs to the outside of your right hand.

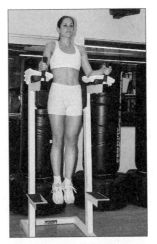

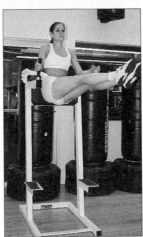

TRAINER'S TIPS

- Don't let your legs rest at the bottom of the movement.
- Let your hips move forward as your legs pass the 90-degree angle.
- Don't swing to gain momentum.
- Control the motion on the way down. Don't just let your legs drop.
- Focus your mind on feeling your abs do the work.
- If you can't get your feet all the way up, just go as high as you can. Your range of motion will improve with work.

■ Hanging Leg Raises with a Cross: Single Leg

DIFFICULTY: 2
LOWER BACK: MODERATE RISK
AREA OF FOCUS: UPPER AND LOWER ABS AND OBLIQUES

STARTING POSITION: Hang from straps or a vertical chair with your legs fully extended.

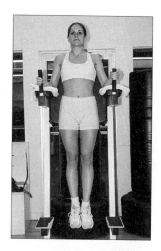

THE MOVE: Use your abs to raise and cross your right leg (knee unlocked) to the outside of your left hand. Then lower your leg back to the starting position. Repeat the movement to the opposite side, bringing your left leg to the outside of your right hand.

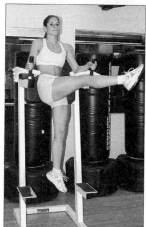

TRAINER'S TIPS

- Don't rest at the bottom of the movement.
- Let your hips move forward as your leg passes the 90-degree angle.
- Don't swing to gain momentum.
- Control the motion on the way down. Don't just let your leg drop.
- Focus your mind on feeling your abs do the work.
- If you can't get your foot all the way up, just go as high as you can. Your range of motion will improve with work.
- The nonworking leg will move slightly forward as the crossing leg reaches the top of the movement.

■ Hanging Knee Raises with a Cross

DIFFICULTY: 3
LOWER BACK: MODERATE RISK
AREA OF FOCUS: UPPER AND LOWER ABS AND OBLIQUES

STARTING POSITION: Hang from straps or a vertical chair with your legs fully extended.

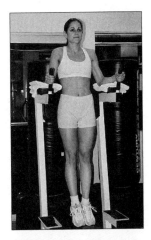

THE MOVE: Use your abs to raise and cross your knees toward your left shoulder. Then lower your legs back to the starting position. Repeat the movement to the opposite side, bringing your knees to your right shoulder.

TRAINER'S TIPS

- Don't let your legs rest at the bottom of the movement.
- Let your hips move forward as your knees pass the 90-degree angle.
- Don't swing to gain momentum.
- Control the motion on the way down. Don't just let your legs drop.
- Focus your mind on feeling your abs do the work.
- If you can't get your knees all the way up, just go as high as you can. Your range of motion will improve with work.

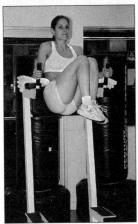

■ Hanging Knee Raises with a Cross: Single Knee

DIFFICULTY: 2

LOWER BACK: MODERATE RISK

AREA OF FOCUS: UPPER AND LOWER ABS AND OBLIQUES

STARTING POSITION: Hang from straps or a vertical chair with your legs fully extended.

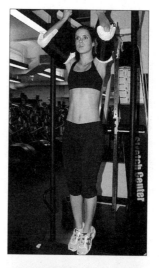

THE MOVE: Use your abs to raise and cross your right knee toward your left shoulder. Then lower your leg back to the starting position. Repeat the movement to the opposite side, bringing your left knee to your right shoulder.

TRAINER'S TIPS

- Don't rest at the bottom of the movement.
- Let your hips move forward as your knee passes the 90-degree angle.
- Don't swing to gain momentum.
- Control the motion on the way down. Don't just let your leg drop.
- Focus your mind on feeling your abs do the work.

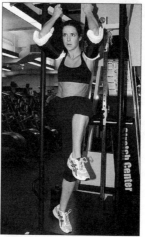

■ Cable Crunches with a Cross

DIFFICULTY: 2
LOWER BACK: LOW RISK
AREA OF FOCUS:
  UPPER ABS AND OBLIQUES

STARTING POSITION: Grab the cable attachment. Kneel facing away from the machine, hips off your heels, holding the attachment with both hands.

THE MOVE: Using the muscles of your abs, bend over and forward, crossing your right shoulder toward your opposite knee while keeping the cable tight and held stationary. Raise your torso back to the starting position. Then bend forward, crossing your left shoulder over your right knee. Repeat to the opposite side.

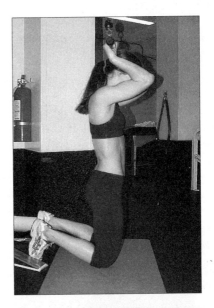

TRAINER'S TIPS

- Raise and lower the weights in a controlled motion. Don't pop up.
- Hold the contraction at the bottom of the movement for a count of two.
- Focus your mind on feeling your abs do the work.

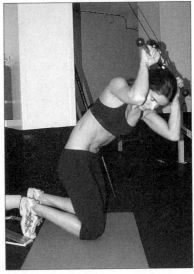

■ P   lts

DIF
LO   OW RISK
AR   S: CORE MUSCLES

STARTING POSITION: Lie flat on your back, knees bent, both feet on the floor, and hands at your side or behind your head.

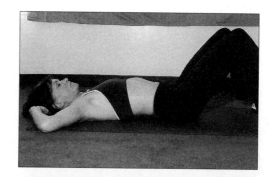

THE MOVE: Rotate your pelvis up and toward your rib cage, pushing the small of your back against the floor. Then let your pelvis rotate back to its normal position so your lower back comes off the floor. Repeat.

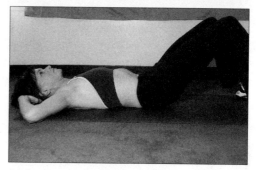

TRAINER'S TIPS

- Don't lift your buttocks off the floor instead of rotating your hips.
- This is a subtle movement. You are using your stomach muscles to rotate your pelvis toward your rib cage to put it in a tilt.

■ Pelvic Rock

DIFFICULTY: 1
LOWER BACK: LOW RISK
AREA OF FOCUS: CORE MUSCLES

STARTING POSITION: Lie flat on your back, knees bent, both feet on the floor, and hands at your side or behind your head.

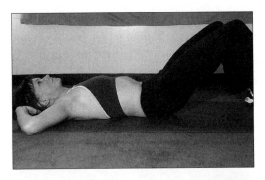

THE MOVE: Rotate your pelvis backward toward your rib cage, pushing the small of your back against the floor. Then rock your pelvis forward so your lower back gently arches. Repeat.

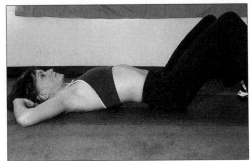

TRAINER'S TIPS

• Feel your deep inner muscles initiate the movement.
• Hold each position for a count of one.

■ Pelvic Clock

DIFFICULTY: 2
LOWER BACK: LOW RISK
AREA OF FOCUS: CORE MUSCLES

STARTING POSITION: Lie flat on your back, knees bent, both feet on the floor, and hands at your side or behind your head.

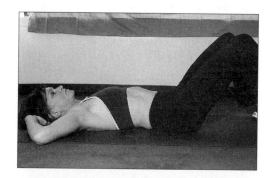

THE MOVE: Imagine that your pelvis is a clock, with twelve o'clock toward your feet, six o'clock toward your chest, three o'clock to your right side, and nine o'clock to your left side. Work your way around the clock, gently hitting all twelve numbers, then repeat in the opposite direction.

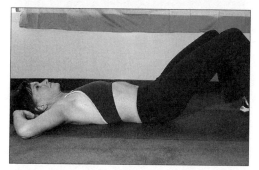

TRAINER'S TIPS

- Don't lift your buttocks off the floor instead of rotating your hips.
- Be precise with each number. This may be frustrating at first, but you will gain better control with practice.
- Breathe. When the movements are small, it is easier to forget to breathe and to hold your breath.

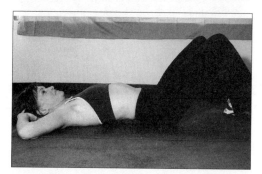

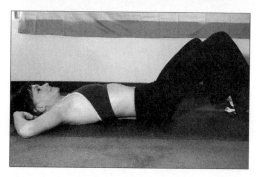

■ Tummy Tucks

DIFFICULTY: 2
LOWER BACK: LOW RISK
AREA OF FOCUS:
  TRANSVERSE ABDOMINIS

STARTING POSITION: Get on all fours, knees under your hips and hands under your shoulders.

THE MOVE: Inhale, then, as you exhale, draw your belly button toward your spine. Inhale and repeat.

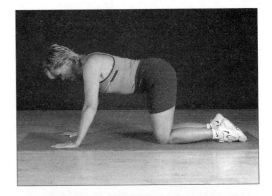

TRAINER'S TIPS

• Focus your mind on pulling your abs up and in.
• Find a steady rhythm with your breathing.
• Focus on pulling in your lower abs at your belly button.

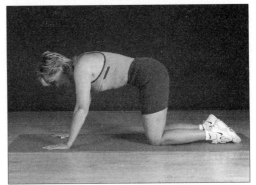

■ Vacuum Pumps

DIFFICULTY: 2
LOWER BACK: LOW RISK
AREA OF FOCUS:
  TRANSVERSE ABDOMINIS

STARTING POSITIONS: (1) On all fours. (2) Kneeling, hands at sides, heels on buttocks, and back straight. (3) Standing, legs slightly bent and hands on thighs.

THE MOVE: Exhale all the air from your body and suck your abdomen up and in as far as you can. Hold for 10 seconds. Relax and repeat.

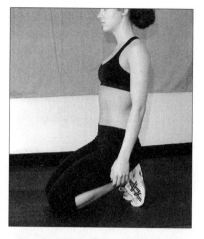

TRAINER'S TIPS

- Focus your mind on pulling your abs up and in.
- Each starting position will get progressively harder, all fours being the easiest and standing the hardest.
- Start out holding each exhalation for 10 seconds and gradually work up to 30 seconds.

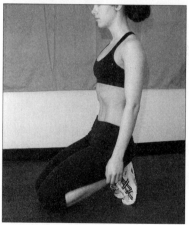

■ Roll-Ups

DIFFICULTY: 2
LOWER BACK: MODERATE RISK
AREA OF FOCUS:
  UPPER AND LOWER ABS

STARTING POSITION: Lie flat on your back, arms at your sides and legs extended straight out.

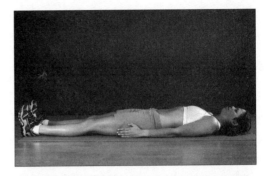

THE MOVE: Roll up vertebra by vertebra until your hands extend out to your toes. Roll back down to the starting position and repeat.

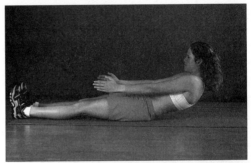

TRAINER'S TIPS

- Keep reaching forward with your arms and keep your heels on the floor at all times.
- Squeeze your buttocks together.
- Let your vertebrae, one by one, follow your arms up and forward.
- Keep your neck lengthened throughout the movement.
- Start the upward movement from the top of your spine and start the downward movement from the bottom of your spine.
- Exhale as you roll up and inhale as you roll down.

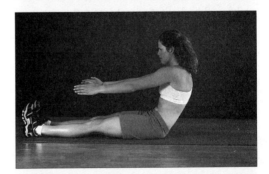

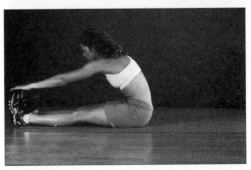

■ Low Twists

DIFFICULTY: 3
LOWER BACK: HIGH RISK
**AREA OF FOCUS: UPPER AND LOWER
  ABS AND OBLIQUES**

STARTING POSITION: In a seated position on the floor, knees bent and feet flat, hold a medicine ball or weight plate and extend it out in front of you. Then lean back, putting tension on your abs.

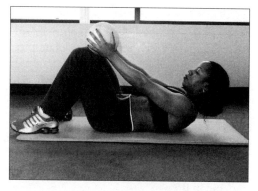

THE MOVE: Twist your torso to the left as you lower the ball down to your hip, then extend the ball out and in front of you. Rotate back to the right, bringing the ball up and over your legs, then down to your hip, extending the ball out and in front of you. Keep alternating sides.

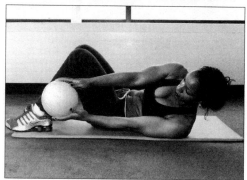

TRAINER'S TIPS

- Find a rhythm in bringing the ball or weight over your knees, then down and out to the side.
- Focus your mind on feeling your abs.
- Keep your neck lengthened.
- Keep your inner core activated to protect your lower back.

■ Air Pumps with a Cross

DIFFICULTY: 2
LOWER BACK: MODERATE RISK
AREA OF FOCUS: UPPER AND LOWER
   ABS AND OBLIQUES

STARTING POSITION: Lie flat on your back with your hands behind your ears and your legs extended, knees over your hips, and your lower legs slightly bent.

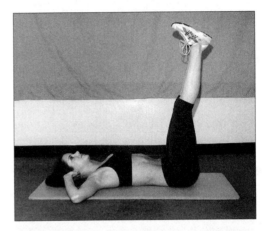

THE MOVE: As you curl your torso up, simultaneously bring your left shoulder and right knee toward each other. Then extend your right leg. Repeat the movement to the opposite side. It's as if you were pedaling a bicycle in the air.

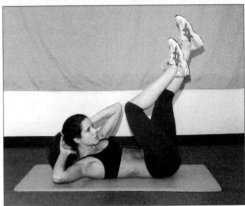

TRAINER'S TIPS

- Focus your mind on feeling your abs do the work.
- Keep your neck lengthened.
- Keep your spine in neutral, being careful not to arch it.
- Extend your lower leg out as you lower your torso.

■ Double Air Pumps

DIFFICULTY: 2
LOWER BACK: MODERATE RISK
**AREA OF FOCUS: UPPER AND LOWER
   ABS AND OBLIQUES**

STARTING POSITION: Lie flat on your back with your hands behind your ears and your legs extended, knees over your hips, and your lower legs slightly bent.

THE MOVE: As you curl your torso up, simultaneously bring both knees toward your chest. As you lower your torso down, extend your lower legs up and out. Repeat.

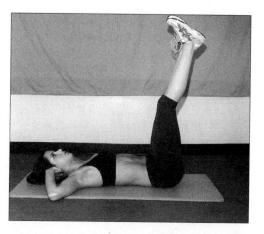

TRAINER'S TIPS

- Focus your mind on feeling your abs do the work.
- Keep your neck lengthened.
- Keep your spine in neutral, being careful not to arch it.
- Find a rhythm in bringing your shoulders and knees together and extending your lower legs as you lower your torso.

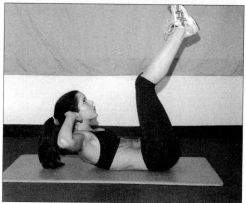

■ Wood Chops: High Cable

DIFFICULTY: 2
LOWER BACK: MODERATE RISK
AREA OF FOCUS: UPPER AND LOWER
 ABS AND OBLIQUES

STARTING POSITION: Stand with your right side facing the weight stack. Grab the handle attachment from the high cable pulley with both hands and bring it to your left shoulder.

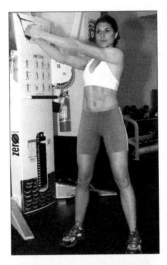

THE MOVE: Rotate and lower your right shoulder toward your left hip. Return to the starting position and repeat to the opposite side.

TRAINER'S TIPS

- Train both sides.
- Use a light weight.
- Focus your mind on feeling your abs do the work.
- Keep your hips facing forward.
- Initiate the movement from your abs—don't pull with your arm.

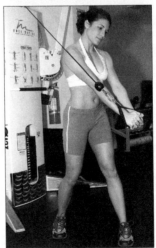

■ Wood Chops: Low Cable

DIFFICULTY: 2
LOWER BACK: MODERATE RISK
AREA OF FOCUS: OBLIQUES AND
   RECTUS ABDOMINIS

STARTING POSITION: Stand with your right side facing the weight stack. Grab the handle attachment from the low cable pulley with both hands at hip height.

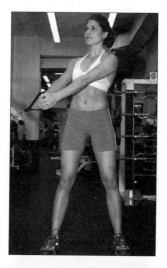

THE MOVE: Rotate your torso as you raise the cable up and diagonally across your body.

TRAINER'S TIPS

- Train both sides.
- Use a light weight.
- Initiate the movement from the center of your body.
- Initiate the movement from your abs, not pulling with your arms.
- Focus your mind on feeling your abs do the work.

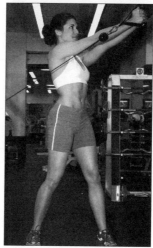

CHAPTER TWENTY-TWO

Area Five:
Core Moves

PREVIEW: *This chapter introduces the exercise ball and moves that train your core-stabilization muscles.*

■ ■ ■

■ On the Ball: Roll-Ins

DIFFICULTY: 2
LOWER BACK: MODERATE RISK
AREA OF FOCUS: LOWER ABS

STARTING POSITION: From a pushup position, have your lower legs and the tops of your feet on top of the ball, placing your hands directly under your shoulders.

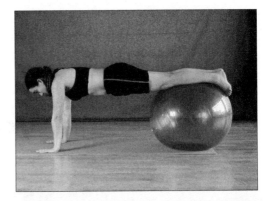

THE MOVE: Bring your knees toward your chest as you slowly roll the ball forward with your ankles and feet. Then straighten your legs, rolling the ball back out to the starting position. Repeat.

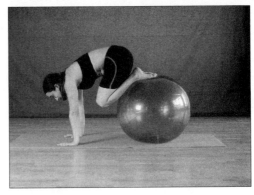

TRAINER'S TIPS

• Keep the ball's movement under control.
• Focus your mind on feeling your lower abs do the work.
• Keep your neck lengthened and look straight down.
• Keep your hands under your shoulders for the entire movement.

■ On the Ball: Reverse Crunches

DIFFICULTY: 2
LOWER BACK: MODERATE RISK
AREA OF FOCUS: LOWER ABS

STARTING POSITION: Lie on your back on top of the ball, placing your feet on the floor. Grab the support bar behind you and raise your feet off the floor until your knees are directly over your hips.

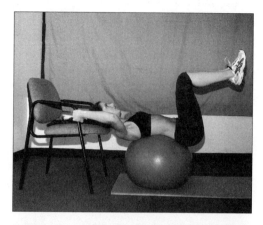

THE MOVE: Curl your knees past your hips, bringing them toward your chest. Repeat.

TRAINER'S TIPS

- Try to raise your hips slightly off the ball as you bring your knees toward your chest.
- Focus your mind on feeling your lower abs do the work.
- Keep your neck lengthened.

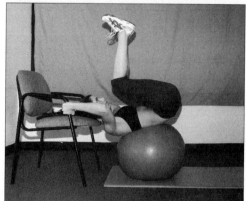

■ On the Ball: Plank Rolls

DIFFICULTY: 2
LOWER BACK: MODERATE RISK
AREA OF FOCUS: OBLIQUES

STARTING POSITION: From a down plank position (see page 257), have your thighs on the ball and your hands directly under your shoulders. To make it more difficult, place your lower legs on top of the ball.

THE MOVE: Using your legs and your oblique muscles, roll the ball to the right as far as you can without losing balance. Then roll the ball back to the starting position and as far to the left as you can. As the ball moves, your legs will get closer to the floor.

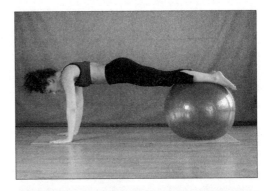

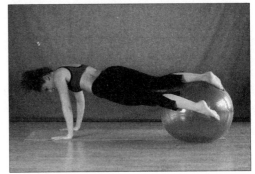

TRAINER'S TIPS

- In this exercise, the goal is to turn the ball in place.
- Focus your mind on your obliques.
- Keep your neck lengthened and look straight down.
- Keep your hands under your shoulders for the entire movement.

■ On the Ball: Plank Twists

DIFFICULTY: 2
LOWER BACK: MODERATE RISK
AREA OF FOCUS: OBLIQUES

STARTING POSITION: From a down plank position (see page 257), have your thighs on the ball. To make it more difficult, place your lower legs or the tops of your feet on top of the ball. Place your hands directly under your shoulders.

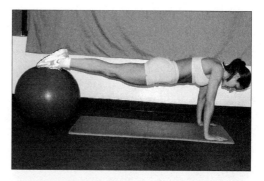

THE MOVE: Keeping your legs on top of the ball, rotate your right hip up to the twelve o'clock position. Then rotate your left hip up to the twelve o'clock position.

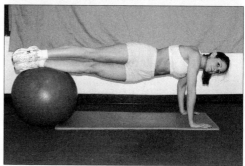

TRAINER'S TIPS

- Try to keep the ball from moving.
- Focus your mind on your obliques.
- Keep your neck lengthened and look straight down.
- Keep your hands under your shoulders for the entire movement.

■ On the Ball: Roll-Outs

DIFFICULTY: 2
LOWER BACK:
  MODERATE TO HIGH RISK
AREA OF FOCUS:
  UPPER AND LOWER ABS

STARTING POSITION: Kneel in front of the ball, placing your hands in a prayer position on top of the ball.

THE MOVE: Roll the ball forward until your arms and shoulders are fully extended. Then roll the ball back to the starting position. Repeat.

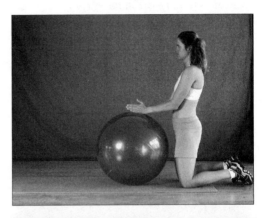

TRAINER'S TIPS

• Focus your mind on your abs.
• Keep your neck lengthened and look straight down.
• Keep your buttocks contracted and your hips stable to protect your lower back.
• Extending your hips forward will make the exercise more difficult.

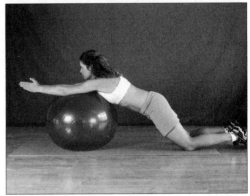

■ On the Ball: Roll-Outs with a Cross

DIFFICULTY: 3
LOWER BACK: HIGH RISK
AREA OF FOCUS: UPPER AND LOWER ABS AND OBLIQUES

STARTING POSITION: Kneel in front of the ball, placing your hands in a prayer position on top of the ball.

THE MOVE: Roll the ball forward and at an angle to your left until your arms and shoulders are fully extended. Then roll the ball back to the starting position and extend the ball out at an angle to your right. Repeat to the other side.

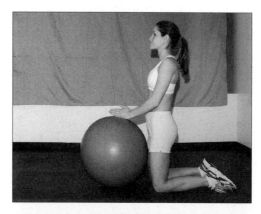

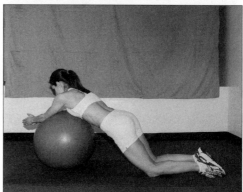

TRAINER'S TIPS

- It's like you're making the letter *V*.
- Focus your mind on your abs.
- Keep your neck lengthened and look straight down.
- Keep your buttocks contracted and your hips stable to protect your lower back.
- Extending your hips forward will make the execise more difficult.

■ On the Ball:
Roll-Ins with a Cross

DIFFICULTY: 3
LOWER BACK: HIGH RISK
AREA OF FOCUS: UPPER AND LOWER
  ABS AND OBLIQUES

STARTING POSITION: From a pushup position, have your lower legs and feet on top of the ball and your hands directly under your shoulders.

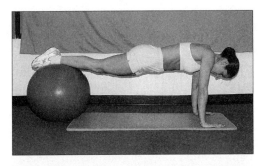

THE MOVE: Bring your knees toward your chest as you slowly roll the ball forward with your ankles and feet. Then extend your legs and the ball back at an angle. Roll the ball back to the starting position and repeat to the other side.

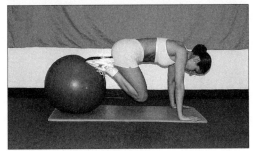

TRAINER'S TIPS

- Draw the letter *V* as you roll the ball back and forth.
- Keep the ball's movement under control.
- Focus your mind on feeling your lower abs do the work.
- Keep your neck lengthened and look straight down.
- Keep your hands under your shoulders for the entire movement.

■ On the Ball: Jackknives

DIFFICULTY: 2
LOWER BACK: MODERATE RISK
AREA OF FOCUS: LOWER ABS

STARTING POSITION: From a pushup position, have the balls of your feet on top of the ball and your arms extended directly under your shoulders. Your body should form a straight line.

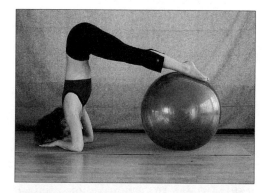

THE MOVE: Use your feet to pull the ball toward your hands as you raise your hips above your hands. Roll the ball back to the starting position and repeat.

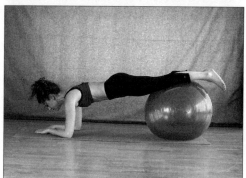

TRAINER'S TIPS

- Keep the ball's movement under control.
- Focus your mind on feeling your lower abs do the work.
- Keep your neck lengthened and in alignment with your spine—don't look up or tuck your chin.
- Keep your elbows under your shoulders for the entire movement.

■ On the Ball: Planks

DIFFICULTY: 2
LOWER BACK: MODERATE RISK
AREA OF FOCUS:
   UPPER AND LOWER ABS

STARTING POSITION: From a down plank position (see page 257), have your feet on top of the ball and your arms extended directly under your shoulders. Your body should form a straight line.

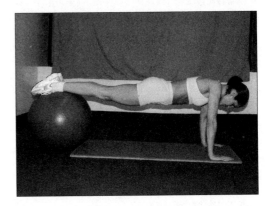

THE MOVE: Hold this position for the prescribed time.

VARIATIONS: You can make this exercise easier by moving your thighs on top of the ball. Or you can make the movement more difficult by putting the balls of your feet on top of the ball.

TRAINER'S TIPS

- Keep the ball from moving.
- Focus your mind on feeling your abs do the work.
- Draw your belly button toward your spine.
- Keep your neck lengthened and in alignment with your spine—don't look up or tuck your chin.
- Keep your hands under your shoulders for the entire movement.

■ On the Ball:
Planks: Hands on Ball

DIFFICULTY: 3
LOWER BACK:
  MODERATE TO HIGH RISK
AREA OF FOCUS:
  UPPER AND LOWER ABS

STARTING POSITION: From a down plank position (see page 257), have your forearms on the ball and your feet on the floor. Your body should form a straight line. You can make this exercise more difficult by putting your hands on the ball and extending your arms.

THE MOVE: Hold this position for the prescribed time.

VARIATION: Rest your feet and knees on the ground.

TRAINER'S TIPS

- Keep the ball from moving.
- Focus your mind on feeling your abs do the work.
- Draw your belly button toward your spine.
- Keep your neck lengthened and in alignment with your spine—don't look up or tuck your chin.

■ On the Ball: Side Bends

DIFFICULTY: 2
LOWER BACK: LOW RISK
AREA OF FOCUS: OBLIQUES

STARTING POSITION: Lie sideways on the ball and scissor your legs wide, with your feet on the floor for support. Place your right hand behind your right ear and your left hand across your waist.

THE MOVE: Raise your torso sideways, bending over your hip. Repeat the movement until you have completed your set. Then switch sides.

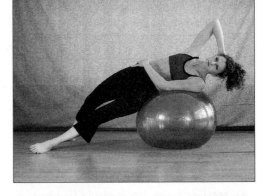

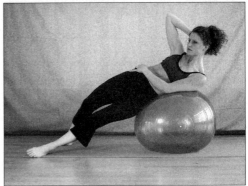

TRAINER'S TIPS

• Keep the ball from moving.
• Think of bringing your rib cage toward your hip.
• Draw your belly button toward your spine.
• Keep your neck lengthened and in alignment with your spine—don't look up or tuck your chin.
• You can make the exercise more difficult by extending your arms over your head.

■ On the Ball:
Torso Corkscrews

DIFFICULTY: 3
LOWER BACK: HIGH RISK
AREA OF FOCUS: OBLIQUES AND
** LOWER-BACK MUSCLES**

STARTING POSITION: Lie sideways on the ball and scissor your legs wide, with your foot on the floor for support. Place your left hand behind your left ear and your right hand on the floor or across the ball.

THE MOVE: Lower and turn your upper body toward the ball. Then raise and rotate your torso back to the starting position. Repeat the movement until you have completed your set. Then switch sides.

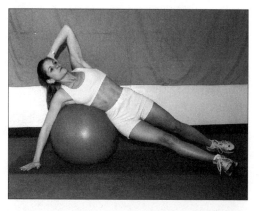

TRAINER'S TIPS

- Don't let the ball move.
- Raise and twist your torso in one motion.
- Draw your belly button toward your spine.
- Keep your neck lengthened and in alignment with your spine—don't look up or tuck your chin.

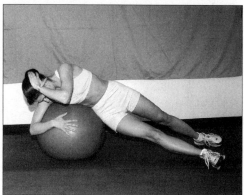

■ On the Ball:
Single-Leg Crunches

DIFFICULTY: 3
LOWER BACK: MODERATE RISK
AREA OF FOCUS:
  UPPER AND LOWER ABS

STARTING POSITION: Sit on top of the ball, your feet on the floor for support. Then slide forward so you're lying on your back and your shoulder blades drop behind the highest part of the ball.

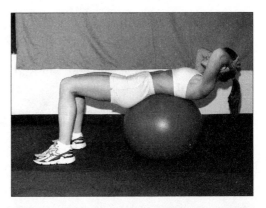

THE MOVE: Curl your upper body forward over the peak of the ball as you raise your left leg so your knee is over your hip. Lower both your torso and leg, then repeat the movement raising your other leg.

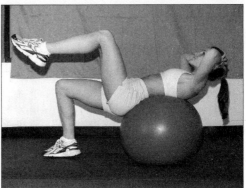

TRAINER'S TIPS

- Don't let the ball move.
- Focus your mind on feeling your abs do the work.
- Make sure you are far enough back on the ball so you have to overcome the angle.

■ On the Ball: Single-Leg Crunches with a Cross

DIFFICULTY: 3
LOWER BACK: MODERATE RISK
AREA OF FOCUS: UPPER AND LOWER ABS AND OBLIQUES

STARTING POSITION: Sit on top of the ball, your feet on the floor for support. Then slide forward so you're lying on your back and your shoulder blades drop behind the highest part of the ball.

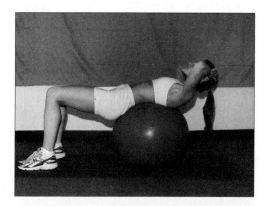

THE MOVE: Curl and cross your right shoulder over the peak of the ball as you raise your left knee toward your right shoulder. Lower both your torso and leg, then repeat the movement to the opposite side.

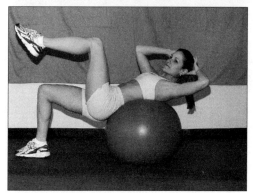

TRAINER'S TIPS

- Keep the ball stable.
- Your leg will move only slightly toward the opposite shoulder.
- Focus your mind on feeling your abs do the work.
- Make sure you are far enough back on the ball so you have to overcome the angle.

■ Basic Trunk Extensions

DIFFICULTY: 1
LOWER BACK: LOW RISK
AREA OF FOCUS: LUMBAR EXTENSORS

STARTING POSITION: Lie on your stomach and rest your forehead on your hands. Your hands should be placed, palms down, on top of each other.

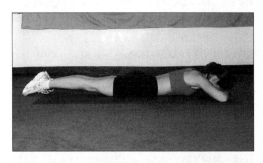

THE MOVE: Lengthening your spine, raise your torso and your head off the floor as high as you can while keeping your hips and feet in place. Lower your body back to the starting position. Repeat.

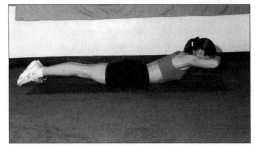

TRAINER'S TIPS

- Throughout the movement, think of lengthening your spine, so the exercise is making you longer and taller.
- Keep your butt and leg muscles tight to protect your lower back.
- Focus on feeling and isolating your lower-back muscles as you raise your torso.

■ Trunk Extensions with Rotation

DIFFICULTY: 2
LOWER BACK: MODERATE RISK
AREA OF FOCUS: LUMBAR EXTENSORS

STARTING POSITION: Lie on your stomach. Looking straight down, place your hands on the back of your head.

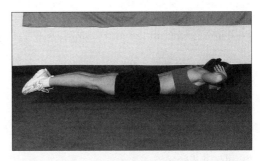

THE MOVE: Lengthening your spine, raise your torso off the floor and rotate your right shoulder up as you turn your head in the same direction. Lower your torso back to the starting position. Repeat the movement, rotating up and to your left.

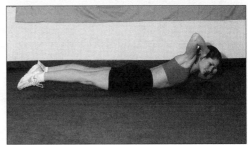

TRAINER'S TIPS

- Throughout the movement, think of lengthening your spine, so the exercise is making you longer and taller.
- Keep your butt and leg muscles tight to protect your lower back.
- Focus on feeling and isolating your lower-back muscles as you raise and turn your torso.
- Keep your neck lengthened.

■ Swimming on All Fours

DIFFICULTY: 2
LOWER BACK: LOW RISK
AREA OF FOCUS: CORE

STARTING POSITION: Get on your hands and knees, with your knees under your hips and your hands under your shoulders.

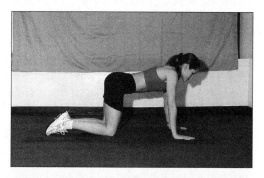

THE MOVE: Simultaneously raise your right arm and left leg so they are parallel with the floor. Hold for a count of three, then lower your arm and leg back to the floor. Repeat the movement with your left arm and right leg.

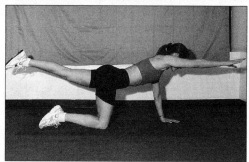

TRAINER'S TIPS

- Focus on keeping your body as straight as a board.
- Don't let your hips sag.
- Keep your neck lengthened and in line with your spine.
- Maintain a steady balance.

■ Swimming on Back

DIFFICULTY: 2
LOWER BACK: MODERATE RISK
AREA OF FOCUS:
  ABDOMINAL MUSCLES

STARTING POSITION: Lie flat on your back with your legs fully extended on the floor and your arms extended over your head.

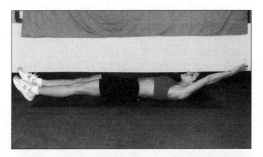

THE MOVE: Simultaneously raise your left arm, your torso, and your right leg. Hold the contraction at the top of movement. Lower your arm, torso, and leg, until they lightly touch the floor. Repeat the movement with your right arm and left leg.

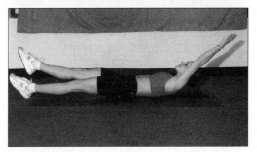

TRAINER'S TIPS

• Before you raise your arm and leg, extend your spine by lengthening the arm and leg you are going to raise.
• Feel the movement initiating from the center of your body.
• Control both the up and the down phases of the movement.
• Keep your neck lengthened and in the proper position.

■ Swimming on Belly

DIFFICULTY: 2
LOWER BACK: MODERATE RISK
AREA OF FOCUS:
  LOWER-BACK MUSCLES

STARTING POSITION: Lie on your stomach with your legs fully extended on the floor and your arms extended over your head. Your head should be facing straight down.

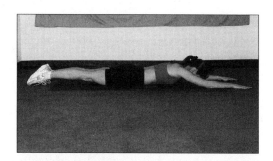

THE MOVE: Simultaneously raise your left arm, your torso, and your right leg. Hold the contraction at the top of the movement. Lower your arm, torso, and leg until they lightly touch the floor. Repeat the movement with your right arm and left leg.

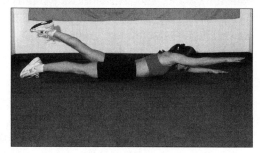

TRAINER'S TIPS

• Before you raise your arm and leg, extend your spine by lengthening the arm and leg you are going to raise.
• Feel the movement initiating from the center of your body.
• Control both the up and the down phases of the movement.
• Keep your neck lengthened and not arched up.

■ Superwomans

DIFFICULTY: 2
LOWER BACK: MODERATE RISK
AREA OF FOCUS:
  LOWER-BACK MUSCLES

STARTING POSITION: Lie flat on your stomach with your legs fully extended on the floor and your arms extended over your head. Your head should be facing straight down.

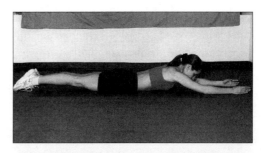

THE MOVE: Simultaneously raise your arms, torso, and legs, as if your were flying. Hold the contraction at the top of the movement. Lower your arms, torso, and legs until they lightly touch the floor. Repeat.

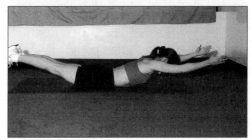

TRAINER'S TIPS

- Before you raise your arms and legs, lengthen your spine by stretching your arms and legs in opposite directions, as if they were being pulled.
- Feel the movement initiating from the center of your body.
- Control both the up and the down phases of the movement.

■ Reverse Superwomans

DIFFICULTY: 2
LOWER BACK: MODERATE RISK
AREA OF FOCUS:
  ABDOMINAL MUSCLES

STARTING POSITION: Lie flat on your back with your legs fully extended on the floor and your arms extended over your head.

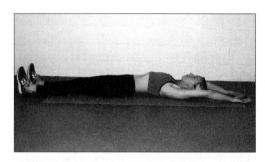

THE MOVE: Simultaneously raise your arms, shoulder blades, and legs off the floor. Hold the contraction at the top of movement. Lower your arms, shoulder blades, and legs until they lightly touch the floor. Repeat.

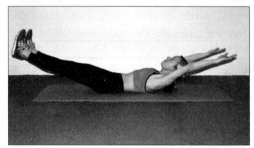

TRAINER'S TIPS

• Before you raise your arms and legs, lengthen your spine by stretching your arms and legs in opposite directions, as if they were being pulled.
• Feel the movement initiating from the center of your body.
• Control both the up and the down phases of the movement.

■ Superwomans with Rotation

DIFFICULTY: 3
LOWER BACK: HIGH RISK
AREA OF FOCUS:
    LOWER-BACK MUSCLES

STARTING POSITION: Lie on your stomach with your legs fully extended on the floor and your arms extended over your head. Your head should be facing straight down.

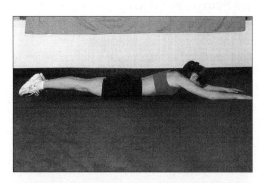

THE MOVE: Simultaneously lengthen your spine and raise your arms, torso, and legs, as if your were flying. Then rotate your right shoulder up as you turn your head in the same direction. Hold the contraction at the top of the movement. Lower your torso back to the starting position and repeat to the opposite side, rotating up and to your left. Lower your arms and legs until they lightly touch the floor. Repeat.

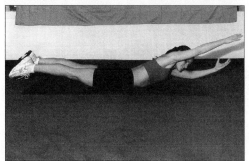

TRAINER'S TIPS

- Before you raise your arms and legs, lengthen your spine by stretching your arms and legs in opposite directions, as if they were being pulled.
- Feel the movement initiating from the center of your body.
- Control both the up and the down phases of the movement.

■ Side Superwomans

DIFFICULTY: 3
LOWER BACK: MODERATE RISK
AREA OF FOCUS: OBLIQUES AND
CORE-STABILIZATION MUSCLES

STARTING POSITION: Lie on your left side with your legs and arms fully extended.

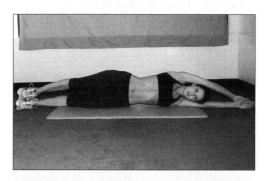

THE MOVE: Simultaneously raise your arms, torso, and legs, as if your were flying on your side. Hold the contraction at the top of the movement. Lower your arms, torso, and legs until they lightly touch the floor. Repeat the movement until you have completed your set. Then switch sides.

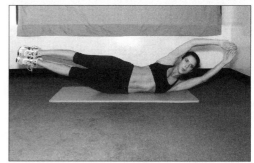

TRAINER'S TIPS

• Before you raise your arms and legs, lengthen your spine by stretching your arms and legs in opposite directions, as if they were being pulled.
• Feel the movement initiating from the center of your body.
• Try to keep your elbows in line with your ears.
• Control both the up and the down phases of the movement.

■ Plank Series

DIFFICULTY: 2
LOWER BACK: LOW RISK
AREA OF FOCUS: CORE

POSITION ONE: DOWN PLANK: Lie on your stomach; raise your body off the floor and support yourself on your forearms (or hands) and your toes. Raise your hips so your body is as straight as a board. Hold for the prescribed time.

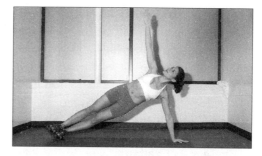

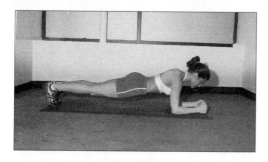

POSITION THREE: UP PLANK: Lie on your back, resting on your forearms (or hands) and your heels. Raise your hips so your body is as straight as a board. Hold for the prescribed time.

POSITION TWO AND THREE: SIDE PLANK: Lie on your left side; rest on your left forearm (or hand) and the outside edge of your left foot. Raise your hips so your body is as straight as a board. Hold for the prescribed time. Repeat on other side.

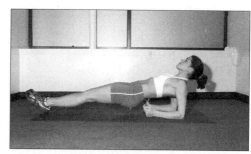

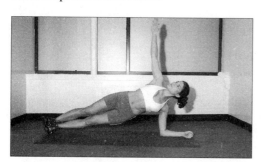

TRAINER'S TIPS

- Focus on keeping your body as straight as a board.
- Don't let your hips sag.
- Keep your neck lengthened and in line with your spine. This will also work your neck-stabilization muscles.

■ Plank: Swimming

DIFFICULTY: 2
LOWER BACK: LOW RISK
AREA OF FOCUS: CORE

STARTING POSITION: Lie on your stomach; raise your body off the floor and support yourself on your hands and your toes. Raise your hips so your body is as straight as a board.

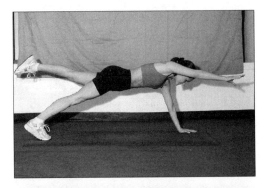

THE MOVE: Simultaneously raise your right arm and left foot off the floor, then lower your foot and arm back to the floor. Repeat with your left arm and right foot.

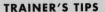

TRAINER'S TIPS

- Focus on keeping your body as straight as a board.
- Don't let your hips sag.
- Keep your neck lengthened and in line with your spine.
- Maintain a steady balance.

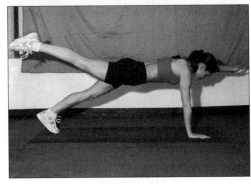

■ Plank: Swinging Gate

DIFFICULTY: 2
LOWER BACK: LOW RISK
AREA OF FOCUS: CORE

STARTING POSITION: Lie on your stomach; raise your body off the floor and support yourself on your hands and the sides of your feet. Raise your hips so your body is as straight as a board.

THE MOVE: Rotate your right hip directly over your left hip, turning your body sideways as you raise your right arm straight in the air, then lower your body back to the starting position. Repeat the movement until you have completed your set. Then switch sides.

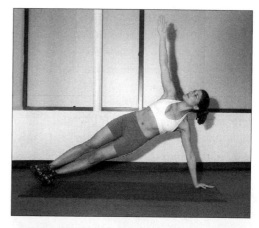

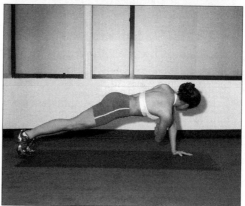

TRAINER'S TIPS

- Focus on keeping your body as straight as a board.
- Don't let your hips sag.
- Keep your neck lengthened and in line with your spine.
- Maintain a steady balance.
- The finishing position is the same as a side plank.

■ Plank: Flutters

DIFFICULTY: 2
LOWER BACK: LOW RISK
AREA OF FOCUS: CORE

STARTING POSITION: Lie on your back, resting on your forearms (or hands) and your heels. Raise your hips so your body is as straight as a board. Your hands should be pointing toward your feet.

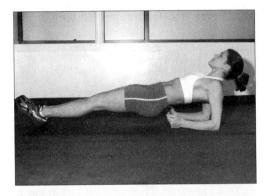

THE MOVE: Raise your left foot and hold it for a count of three, then lower it. Repeat with your right foot.

TRAINER'S TIPS

- Focus on keeping your body as straight as a board.
- Don't let your hips sag.
- Keep your neck lengthened and in line with your spine.
- Maintain a steady balance.

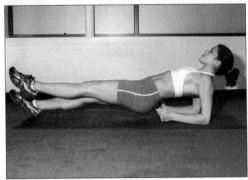

■ Sun Salutations

DIFFICULTY: 2
LOWER BACK: MODERATE RISK
AREA OF FOCUS: CORE

STARTING POSITION: Stand with your legs spread wider than shoulder-width and your arms extended above your head.

THE MOVE: Bend at your waist and reach down and touch the floor in front of your toes, extending and keeping your torso straight and moving as one unit. Straighten back to the starting position.

VARIATION: As you lower your torso, angle your body over your right leg, then return to the starting position. Repeat on the opposite side.

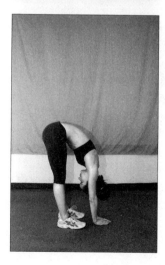

TRAINER'S TIPS

- Focus on keeping your body as straight as a board.
- Keep your neck lengthened and in line with your spine.
- Maintain a steady balance.
- Initiate the movement from your lower back and abs.
- Keep your inner core activated throughout the exercise.

■ Inchworm

DIFFICULTY: 2
LOWER BACK: MODERATE RISK
AREA OF FOCUS: CORE

STARTING POSITION: Lie on your stomach and raise your body off the floor, supporting yourself on your hands and your toes. Raise your hips so your body is as straight as a board.

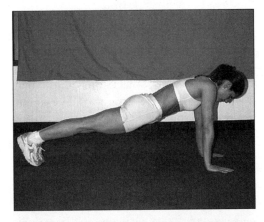

THE MOVE: Walk your feet up toward your hands as far as you can. Then walk your hands back out to the plank position. Repeat by walking your feet up to your hands, then walking your hands out to the plank pushup position. Continue to repeat the movement.

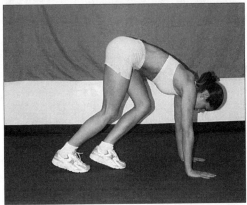

TRAINER'S TIPS

- Focus on keeping your body as straight as a board.
- Keep your neck lengthened and in line with your spine.
- Maintain a steady balance.
- Keep the motion fluid.
- You will move forward with each repetition, so give yourself room to crawl.

■ Ankle Reaches

DIFFICULTY: 2
LOWER BACK: MODERATE RISK
AREA OF FOCUS: CORE

STARTING POSITION: Lie on your stomach, arms and hands at your sides.

THE MOVE: Reach your arms back and up as you bend your lower legs up, bringing your ankles above your knees. Try to touch your hands to your ankles. Return to the starting position and repeat.

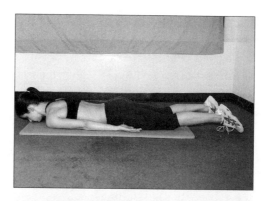

TRAINER'S TIPS

- Keep your neck lengthened and in line with your spine.
- Maintain a steady balance.
- Keep the motion fluid.
- Reach back and up with your arms as you bring your lower legs forward.

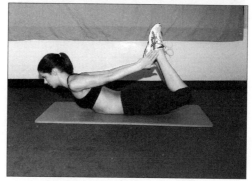

■ Back Extensions: Roman Chair

DIFFICULTY: 2
LOWER BACK: MODERATE RISK
AREA OF FOCUS:
LOWER-BACK MUSCLES

STARTING POSITION: Secure yourself in a Roman chair, feet under the supports. Make sure the chair is adjusted so your waist can bend completely forward.

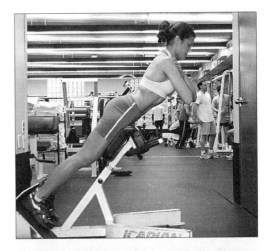

THE MOVE: Bend forward through a full range of motion, making sure your spine and neck stay in alignment. Raise your torso back to the starting position, your spine neutral, not curved or rounded. Repeat.

TRAINER'S TIPS

- Keep your neck lengthened and in line with your spine.
- You can place your hands behind your head or across your chest, or hold a weight plate.
- Keep the motion fluid.
- Don't hyperextend your back.

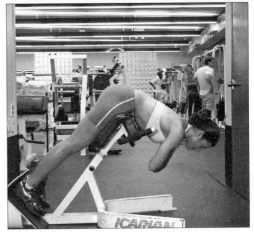

■ Back Extensions with a Twist: Roman Chair

DIFFICULTY: 2
LOWER BACK: MODERATE RISK
AREA OF FOCUS:
 LOWER-BACK MUSCLES

STARTING POSITION: Secure yourself in a Roman chair, feet under the supports. Make sure the chair is adjusted so your waist can bend completely forward.

THE MOVE: Bend forward through a full range of motion, making sure your spine and neck stay in alignment. As you raise your torso back to the starting position, rotate your right shoulder up, twisting your torso in that direction. Alternate the direction of the twist with each repetition.

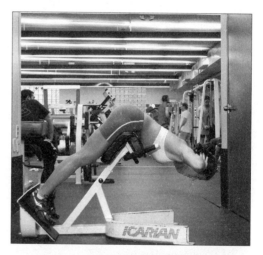

TRAINER'S TIPS

- Let your head turn in the direction of the twist.
- Keep your neck lengthened and in line with your spine.
- You can place your hands behind your head or across your chest, or hold a weight plate.
- Keep the motion fluid.
- Don't hyperextend your back.

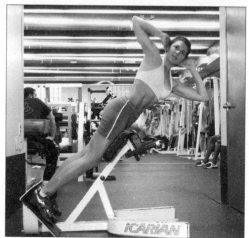

CONTRIBUTORS

BRETT BRUNGARDT is the strength and conditioning coach at the University of Washington. He has been involved in fitness for over twenty years. He has a master's degree in exercise science from the University of Houston. He has been the strength and conditioning coach at the University of Houston, the University of Wyoming, and the University of Kentucky. He was also the strength and conditioning coach for the Dallas Mavericks in the NBA. He is a certified strength and conditioning specialist with the National Strength and Conditioning Association.

MIKE BRUNGARDT is the strength and conditioning coach for the two-time NBA champion San Antonio Spurs. He's been a fitness consultant and personal trainer for over twenty years. He is president of the NBA Strength Coaches Association.

BRYON HOLMES has been involved in all aspects of the health and fitness field. He is one of the country's top experts in lower-back care and rehabilitation. He has authored over forty articles and abstracts on lower-back care. He has a B.S. and M.S. in exercise physiology from the University of Florida.

DEBBIE HOLMES is a fitness educator, teacher, and personal trainer. She is a member of the American College of Sports Medicine and the American Council on Exercise. She has a B.S. and M.S. in health and exercise education from the University of Florida. She is the owner and operator of the Medex Health Club and the Estes Park Health and Racquet Club, both in Estes Park, Colorado.

DAVE JOHNSON is a personal trainer and writer. He has been training clients in the New York City area for ten years. He lives in New York City.

MARTIN KAMMLER is a personal trainer in New York City. He has a master's degree in sports science from the University of Bochum, in Germany. He has worked extensively in sports clubs and rehabilitation centers. Martin has worked with some of Germany's top athletes as well as teaching a variety of classes, including spinning, Aqua-Power, and weight training. Along with training clients in New York, Martin develops and designs fitness equipment. You can reach Martin at Kammlerfitness.com.

STEVEN WILDE is a personal trainer and fitness consultant in Los Angeles, California. He has been involved in sports and fitness for more than twenty years. He has worked with a wide variety of clients, from celebrities and business professionals to senior citizens and kids.

MODELS

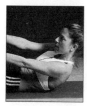

KATIE CAMERON is an actress. She has appeared in dozens of plays in New York City and at regional theaters.

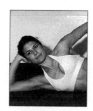

CLAUDIA HICKEY is a personal trainer at New York Sports Clubs. She was an NCAA athlete in softball and track at the University of Virginia. She lives in New York City.

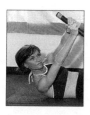

KENDRA FRANCIS is serious about working out and the martial arts. She lives in Denver, Colorado.

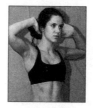

ELISABETH HOWERS is a personal trainer and an actor. She is studying theater at Marymount College in New York.

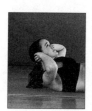

RANDIA HAZLETT is a workout enthusiast. She has a degree in social work from Colorado State University and a dog named Panchi. She lives with her husband, Cody, in Fort Collins, Colorado.

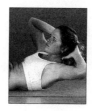

LAURA KATERS is a personal trainer, a writer, and an artist. She lives in Fort Collins, Colorado.

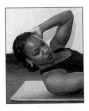 **JEHINA MALIK** is a personal trainer at New York Sports Clubs and a professional bodybuilder. She lives in New York City.

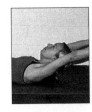 **LEA VANSICKLE** works out at her vintage-clothing store, Mint. She lives in Fort Collins, Colorado.

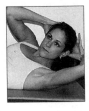 **FELICIA MANNINO** is a personal trainer at New York Sports Clubs. She is getting a dual master's degree in nursing and health administration. She can be contacted at feliciamannino@hotmail.com. She lives in New York City.

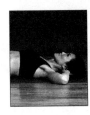 **KISHA WATANABE** is a workout enthusiast. She lives in Denver, Colorado.

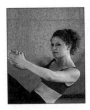 **TRACY MARX** is a writer and wannabe supermodel. She lives in New York City.

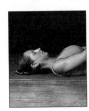 **KALI LORING WEIL** loves to do yoga and be active. She lives in Fort Collins, Colorado.

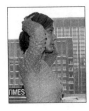 **ANDREA QUAST** is a workout and fitness enthusiast. She lives in Fort Collins, Colorado.

INDEX

Page numbers in italics *refer to illustrations.*

ABOUT THE AUTHOR

KURT BRUNGARDT is the author or co-author of seven fitness books, including the bestselling *The Complete Book of Abs*. He has appeared on the *Today* show, *20/20*, and *Good Morning America*. He has been featured in such major publications as *The New York Times*, *The London Times*, *Men's Health*, *Self*, *Shape*, and *Details*. He is also the writer and host of the bestselling video *Abs of Steel for Men*. As a personal trainer, Brungardt has worked with a wide variety of clients, ranging from adolescents to senior citizens, corporate executives to celebrities, beginners to world-class athletes. His other books include *The Complete Book of Butt and Legs*, *The Complete Book of Shoulders and Arms*, *3-Minute Abs*, *Essential Abs*, *Essential Arms*, and *Essential Chest*. His most recent video, *Action Sports Camp*, is an imaginative and fun workout for kids.